Capturing Nursing History

About the Editors

In her role as Professor of Nursing at the Lienhard School of Nursing, Pace University, **Sandra B. Lewenson, EdD, RN, FAAN,** brings nursing's rich history into the classroom. She teaches an online nursing history course to both undergraduate and graduate nursing students making history accessible and part of their educational experience. Dr. Lewenson weaves her love of nursing history into all the courses she teaches, including courses on decision making, nursing education, and nursing research. She recently served as the President of the American Association for the History of Nursing and continues to be actively involved in this organization. Her research interests include nursing's historical political activity, the integration of nursing history into the curriculum, the evidence of *nursism* and its influence on the profession, and the history of nursing education in the United States. She has been the recipient of the Outstanding Scholarship and Research Award from Teachers College, Columbia University, inducted into the Hall of Fame of the Alumni Association of Hunter College, and received the American Association for the History of Nursing Lavinia Dock Award for Historical Scholarship and Research in Nursing. Dr. Lewenson is a Fellow of the American Academy of Nursing and a member of Sigma Theta Tau International Honor Society.

Throughout her career, noted nurse historian and Professor Emerita from University of Connecticut, **Eleanor Krohn Herrmann, EdD, RN, FAAN,** has been devoted to preserving nursing history and designing nursing curriculum for future generations. Both of her interests took her to Central and South America where she was instrumental in establishing the curriculum of Ecuador's first university-level school of nursing under the auspices of Project Hope. Since 1969, she has had an ongoing relationship with the nursing profession in Belize, Central America, as well as with several other countries in this area of the world. Dr. Herrmann has served on the faculties of several universities, including Yale and the Universities of Connecticut, Wyoming, Colorado, Syracuse, and Cornell. Dr. Herrmann has served as president of the prestigious American Association for the History of Nursing, and is the author of several articles, books, and monographs on various aspects of nursing history. One of her most noted works is the *History of Belizean Nursing Education,* published in 1985 as the *Origins of Tomorrow.* Dr. Herrmann has been the recipient of several awards in nursing, such as Yale University School of Nursing's Annie W. Goodrich Award for Excellence in Teaching and the Connecticut Nurses Association's Josephine A. Dolan Award. She is a Fellow of the American Academy of Nursing and a member of Sigma Theta Tau International Honor Society. For many years, Dr. Herrmann has been engaged in curating the University of Connecticut's historic Dolan Collection, and she continues to mentor nurse historians throughout the world.

Capturing Nursing History

A Guide to Historical Methods in Research

Sandra B. Lewenson, EdD, RN, FAAN
Eleanor Krohn Herrmann, EdD, RN, FAAN
Editors

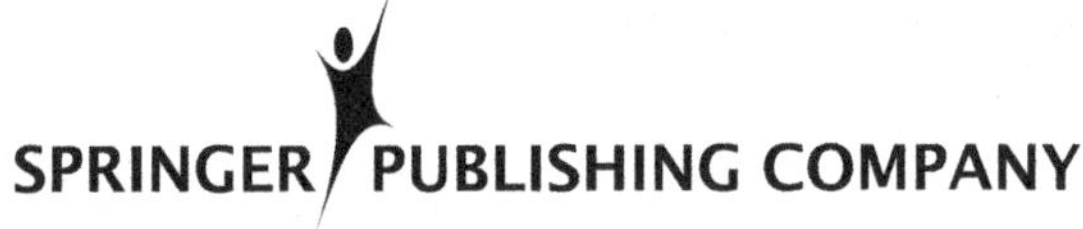

New York

Springer Publishing Company, LLC
11 West 42nd Street
New York, NY 10036
www.springerpub.com

Acquisitions Editor: Allan Graubard
Project Manager: Carol Cain
Cover design: Joanne E. Honigman
Composition: Apex Publishing, LLC

07 08 09 10/ 5 4 3 2 1

Library of Congress Cataloging-in-Publication Data

Capturing nursing history : a guide to historical methods in research / Sandra B. Lewenson, Eleanor Krohn Herrmann, editors.
p. ; cm.
Includes bibliographical references and index.
ISBN-13: 978-0-8261-1566-9 (alk. paper)
ISBN-10: 0-8261-1566-7 (alk. paper)
1. Nursing—Historiography. 2. Nursing—Research—Methodology. I. Lewenson, Sandra. II. Herrmann, Eleanor Krohn.
[DNLM: 1. Historiography. 2. History of Nursing. 3. Nursing Research—methods. WY 11.1 C254 2008]
RT31.C37 2008
610.73—dc22

2007035620

Printed in the United States of America by Bang Printing.

Contents

Contributors

Nettie Birnbach, EdD, RN, FAAN
Professor Emerita
College of Nursing
State University of New York at Brooklyn
Brooklyn, New York
United States

Nerrisa Bonifacio, RN, BSN
Master of Science in Nursing Program
University of British Columbia School of Nursing
Vancouver, British Columbia
Canada

Geertje Boschma, RN, PhD
Associate Professor
School of Nursing
University of British Columbia
Vancouver, British Columbia
Canada

Joy Buck, PhD, RN
Associate Professor
West Virginia University School of Nursing and the Robert C. Byrd Health Sciences Center, Eastern Division,
Morgantown, West Virginia
United States

Cynthia Anne Connolly, PhD, RN, PNP
Assistant Professor
Graduate Entry Prespecialty in Nursing
Assistant Professor in the History of Medicine and Science—YSM
Yale School of Nursing
New Haven, Connecticut
United States

Patricia D'Antonio, RN, PhD, FAAN
Associate Professor
Associate Director, Barbara Bates Center for the Study of the History of Nursing
University of Pennsylvania School of Nursing
Philadelphia, Pennsylvania
United States

Julie A. Fairman, PhD, FAAN, RN
Class of 1940 Bicentennial Term Associate Professor of Nursing, and Director of the Barbara Bates Center for the Study of the History of Nursing
University of Pennsylvania School of Nursing
Philadelphia, Pennsylvania
United States

Janet L. Fickeissen, RN, MSN
Executive Secretary
American Association for the History of Nursing
Lanoka Harbor, New Jersey
United States

Sonya J. Grypma, PhD, RN
Associate Professor
Trinity Western University
Langley, British Columbia
Canada

Christine Hallett, PhD, RGN
Senior Lecturer
School of Nursing, Midwifery, and Social Work
Director
The UK Centre for the History of Nursing and Midwifery
University of Manchester
Manchester, M13 9PL
England

Joan E. Lynaugh, RN, PhD, FAAN
Professor Emeritus
University of Pennsylvania School of Nursing
Philadelphia, Pennsylvania
United States

Keith C. Mages, MSN, MLS, RN
University of Pennsylvania School of Nursing
Doctoral Program
Philadelphia, Pennsylvania
United States

Florence Melchior, PhD, RN
Nursing Instructor
Division of Health Studies
Medicine Hat College
Medicine Hat, Alberta
Canada

Erica Roberts, RN, BSN
Master of Science in Nursing Program
University of British Columbia School of Nursing
Vancouver, British Columbia
Canada

Margaret Scaia, RN, BSN, MN
Senior Instructor
University of Victoria
Victoria, British Columbia
Canada

Jean C. Whelan, PhD, RN
Adjunct Assistant Professor of Nursing
University of Pennsylvania School of Nursing
Philadelphia, Pennsylvania
United States

Foreword

Because historians are actually the creators of the past and not merely its recorders, we know it is vital that we approach our work seriously and use the best tools we can find. In *Capturing Nursing History,* we now have a major asset for ourselves and for our successors. All of us are in debt to the editors and authors who conceived of and created this invaluable text. Scholars will be enabled and scholarship will be enhanced because this book is now available.

And, although long needed, it couldn't come at a better time. For, although Janet Wilson James told us in 1984 there were "signs of life and thought reviving" in the history of nursing, we knew we had a long way to go. Nearly 25 years later, scholarship in the history of nursing is, indeed, very much alive and full of thought. Patricia D'Antonio (Chapter 2) reminds us that we have, over time, "told many fascinating and important stories that have created collective meanings and memories for a quite disparate group of professionals." But, there is much to do, many more avenues to explore, and many more audiences to reach. We need to be open to the ways people relate to the past and reach out to them with our stories.

At the same time, it is crucial that we hold fast to our investment and belief in scholarship and in the integrity of our historical products. For it is our history, our known and ordered past, that makes it possible to imagine new goals and envision a collective future for nursing. *Capturing Nursing History* is an outstanding and unique guide to that integrity and best scholarship. It is a good time to be a historian.

Joan E. Lynaugh, PhD, FAAN
Professor Emeritus,
School of Nursing, University of Pennsylvania

REFERENCE

James, J. W. (1984). Writing and rewriting nursing history: A review essay. *Bulletin of the History of Medicine, 58,* 568–584.

Preface

Our interest in writing *Capturing Nursing History: A Guide to Historical Methods in Research* stemmed from our own work in this area. Based on our experiences in historiography, we felt a need to help others develop the skills needed to capture nursing's history. We also wanted to garner the wisdom of those who engage in historiography and share it with a wider audience. We approached this book from the standpoint of how one goes about studying history, specifically, nursing history. We began by examining how we became interested in nursing history and historiography. We found that we both began by questioning the world around us, searching for meaning behind a particular phenomenon, event, period, or place. The question, "Why?" led to a myriad of other questions that often left us dazed at the prospect of how to approach a historiographic study. When beginning a historical research project, we had to stop and ask ourselves, "Where do I start?" and "What do I need to consider when doing historical research?" These are two important questions that led us to develop the manuscript for this book.

We felt that to help others study nursing history and engage in historiography, a book such as *Capturing Nursing History: A Guide to Historical Methods in Research* would be an essential tool. There are few avenues that support the nurse historian in doing historical research and even fewer mentors that can point the way. Certainly, the American Association for the History of Nursing (AAHN), provides much needed support for nurse historians who undertake this type of research. The AAHN augments the doctoral programs in nursing that permit historical dissertations and historians who share their craft with others as a personal and professional need to understand historical antecedents to various phenomena. Other support for nurse historians comes from the various centers that have opened in the past 20 years or more, such as the Bellevue Alumnae Center for Nursing History at the New York State Foundation of Nurses; the Barbara Bates Center for the Study of the History of Nursing at the University of Pennsylvania; the Center for Nursing

Historical Inquiry at the University of Virginia Health Sciences Center; the Midwest Nursing History Research Center at the University of Illinois, Chicago; the Archives of Nursing Leadership at the University of Connecticut School of Nursing; and the Thomas J. Dodd Research Center. These resources and others, which appear on the AAHN Web site (http://aahn.org/) and in the appendix of the book, provide guidance in historical research.

Yet, even with these supports, we saw that a void exists in support for the budding and experienced nurse historian. Very often researchers worked solo and only saw their own professional history, only acknowledged what they experienced, and could not make connections with others. While there are some supports, such as those mentioned in the previous paragraph, and some articles and chapters in books that address the historical research method (these can also be found on the AAHN Web site), few (if any) texts exist that contain the collected wisdom about doing historical research in nursing. This book hopes to augment the supports that currently exist and provide much needed guidance to all levels of nurse historians.

Capturing Nursing History: A Guide to Historical Methods in Research provides a form of mentorship to the nurse historian. We designed the book to assist individuals interested in doing historical research in nursing by offering the knowledge and insights of experts who have conducted this type of work before. We asked noted nurse historians to share their ideas about the research they do in nursing history.

Each chapter provides an aspect of historical research that historians need to address. The contributors write about a variety of approaches to historiography and share their insights and wisdom. They describe how they approach their investigations and the steps they take in doing historical research. The work represents a culmination of many years of experience, practice, and reflection. Readers hear each contributor's unique voice as they explore the meaning of historical research.

The book includes topics such as how to go about doing a historiography including how to approach biographical research and oral histories. Other topics include the many theoretical frameworks that one can use in historical research and the ethical guidelines and standards that may assist the researcher. The book examines how one does historical research in international settings and how to use artifacts, information rarely found in books containing historical methods. Questions about primary sources, archives, data searches, and institutional review board concerns are also addressed. Nurse historians constantly look for funding sources that will support their historical research and this, too, can be found in this text.

Case studies throughout the chapters illustrate the how, what, where, why, and when historical research is used in nursing. These case studies make the research process more user-friendly and attainable by giving examples that historians have experienced before. Within the case studies, readers may identify with some of the methodological issues that arise and learn how the contributing authors dealt with these issues.

Capturing Nursing History: A Guide to Historical Methods in Research serves as an essential textbook for new and seasoned nurse historians and can serve as a supplement for nursing research courses on both the graduate and undergraduate levels. The book hopes to answer the two questions raised earlier, "Where do I start?" and "What do I need to consider when doing historical research?" In fact, anyone interested in historical research or nursing history can use this book, whether as a simple "how to" or as a general resource for research methods, including those who work in other disciplines. For example, someone interested in studying the history of their institution will find this book as useful as someone interested in completing a historical dissertation in nursing. Hospitals, schools, and state nurses' associations planning to write historical accounts about their organizations and the individuals who had an impact on them will also find this book a useful tool to help them through the process. Likely, the members of the American Association for the History of Nursing (AAHN) as well as other similar professional organizations will also be interested in this work.

Each chapter contributes to the understanding of approaching nursing history and historiography. Yet, the book can be read in any order, and each chapter can be read as a stand-alone. In nursing history courses or in research courses, faculty can assign various chapters (as well as the whole text) to support student learning. Researchers can also use this text to guide them through the process of historical research. We encourage readers to pick and choose the sections that support their research and their questions as they arise during their work.

Chapter 1, "Why Do Historical Research?" explores the rationale for doing historical research. One needs to value history in order to want to study history. This chapter examines what you need to start a historical research project. It also addresses how one becomes a nurse historian. Lewenson and Herrmann reflect on the past to understand how historians become historians—what in their past influenced them to seek out historical evidence to explain the subject under investigation. Finally, this chapter addresses how to engage others in using, reading, and doing historical research. How we integrate history into the fabric of the profession and the broader society is crucial and thus relies on historians to encourage others to support this type of research design in nursing.

In Chapter 2, "Conceptual and Methodological Issues in Historical Research," *Nursing History Review* editor and nurse historian, Patricia D'Antonio, presents her thoughts on some of the conceptual and methodological issues surrounding historical research. In her chapter, she explores five conceptual issues including the "interconnectedness of variables or concepts, the manipulation of such variables or concepts in time and place, contextualization, judgment...and a tolerance for ambiguity" (D'Antonio, in press). She also presents methodological issues that historians often struggle with identifying them as reading, representation, and writing. D'Antonio uses historical research to illustrate each issue thus making the theoretical eminently practical. She explores the ways in which historians may approach historical research and challenges us to start reading, doing historical research, and writing.

Where to begin a historical study can keep many researchers from moving forward. Chapter 3, "Doing Historical Research," describes a way to approach historical research and begin the process. Historical research, however, cannot be completed in a linear fashion. Instead, the data, the questions, the sources, and a myriad of other factors interact and serve as a guide to the steps one takes during the research process. Steps leading to a final product in research may be artificial, yet, they often help in understanding the process. Lewenson uses her current research project to illustrate the approach she uses in historical research. This chapter presents a pragmatic way to look at this type of research design and provides a guide to support all levels of historical researchers.

In Chapter 4, "Using Frameworks in Historical Research," historian Joy Buck shows how historians can use frameworks to shape their historical investigations. She explores the use of a social, cultural, and policy framework and includes examples of studies that use each of these frameworks. She provides a discussion that assists historians to identify the rationale for using frameworks and some of the possibilities that frameworks can afford the researcher. Of special interest is Buck's (2004) use of portions of her previously published work on the American hospice movement. Here, Buck applies a social policy framework when she investigated the establishment of the hospice movement in the United States. By doing so, Buck illustrates how a framework directs the historian to ask relevant questions and seek appropriate data that, in her case, contained social and policy content.

Chapter 5 contains a reprinted article by Sonya Grypma (2005) titled, "Critical Issues in the Use of Biographic Methods in Nursing," which was first published in *Nursing History Review.* This important chapter raises several issues related to a "new historiography" and its application in a biographical investigation. We liked the article when we first read it and continue to find value in the author's ideas. Grypma addresses important theoretical issues in doing biographical research and therefore needed to be part of this book.

Nurse historians, Geertje Boschma, Margaret Scaia, Nerrisa Bonifacio, and Erica Roberts provide an interesting approach to examining the use of oral histories. In Chapter 6, "Oral History Research," the authors explore some of the benefits of this design, such as using subjects who may not be part of the written record and therefore would be typically excluded from historical data and critique. Each one of the contributors offers insight into the issues surrounding oral histories and refers to their own work in this area. They explore some of the unique features of oral history, such as examining the issues of memory and subjectivity, selection and sampling, consent, and therapeutic and transformative potential. They also look at how oral history can inform nursing practice and thus be a very relevant and vital historical research design.

In Chapter 7, "Reflections on Researcher Subjectivity and Identity in Nursing History," nurse historians Geertje Boschma, Sonya Grypma, and Florence Melchior explore their experiences while working on oral histories and biographies. Each author tells their story interjecting how subjectivity may have influenced the research process. The authors present three philosophical perspectives—post-structuralist, phenomenological, and epistemological—to facilitate a thoughtful analysis of their research experience. Boschma uses a post-structuralist perspective to reflect on the work she did collecting oral histories about families experiencing mental illness. Grypma uses a phenomenological perspective to reflect on the research she did on the Canadian missionary work in China. Finally, Melchior reflects on the biographical work she did using an epistemological perspective.

Using her experiences of doing historical research in nursing in both Central and South America, Eleanor Krohn Herrmann wrote Chapter 8, "Historical Research in Developing Countries." In this chapter, Herrmann asks the reader to examine their rationale for undertaking a historical investigation in a developing country. Often the reason one chooses such a venue may relate to one,'s cultural background, or a need to provide culturally sensitive care, or because of a work experience, such as the Peace Corps. Doing historical research in a developing country is very much like doing historical research anywhere, yet, additional work needs to be done in order to be successful. Referring back to her own experiences, Herrmann considers what needs to happen before you travel to the far off corners of the world. For example, you need to check out the availability of primary source materials about your subject, and what, if any, additional documentation you need to bring with you when you visit that location. You also need to arrange how you will do the research, considering things such as use of computers, use of electricity, copiers, and other such amenities that very often we take for granted in countries that are more industrialized than the one you may be visiting. Herrmann draws from her experience providing readers with a down-to-earth process to use when undertaking historical research in a developing country.

Keith C. Mages and Julie A. Fairman open Chapter 9, "Working With Primary Sources: An Overview," with a diary entry by Mary V. Clymer, dated August 4, 1888. Clymer kept a diary documenting her hospital ward experience as a student at the Training School for Nurses at the Hospital of the University of Pennsylvania. Mages and Fairman's use of this primary source document provides an example in which to discuss various issues related to the use of primary source material. Mages and Fairman define and distinguish what primary and secondary source materials refer to and how both are essential to the historical research process. They include useful information about where and how to access online and other primary source material. Throughout the chapter, they use Clymer's diary as an example to explain the many facets of primary source materials. Included in this chapter is the more recent concern about the use of the 1996 Health Insurance Portability and Accountability Act (HIPAA). Here again, Mages and Fairman use Clymer's diary to explain this legal issue that historians must now address.

In Chapter 10, "'The Truth About the Past?' The Art of Working With Archival Material," historian Christine Hallett raises questions about the *truth* and what it means to the historian in search of the truth. The author questions whether there are multiple truths, and, if so, can they be found in the archival materials. Hallett explores how archives reflect upon and influence the research questions. She presents some of the official and unofficial archival collections found in developed countries, using the British National Archives and the National Archives of Australia as two examples of official archives. Hallett also explains that interpretation of the materials relies in part on the historian being able to reflect on their own "pre-existing" assumptions.

Noted for her work *Turn-of-the-Century Nursing Artifacts* (2006), author and nurse historian Eleanor Krohn Herrmann writes about the use of artifacts in Chapter 11, "About Artifacts." In this chapter, Herrmann explores the use of artifacts in historical research. For example, one of the benefits of using this type of source material is the "sense of continuity" one has with a three-dimensional object. Understanding how to acquire such objects, how to value them, and then how to determine their age are presented in this chapter. Herrmann explains how these objects further the understanding of nursing and provide valuable sources for us to use in the research design.

Ethical issues in nursing history require historians to step back and think about the work they do. Chapter 12, "Ethical Guidelines and Standards of Professional Conduct," includes a reprint of two important documents, *Ethical Guidelines for the Nurse Historian* and *Standards of Professional Conduct for Historical Inquiry in Nursing* (Birnbach, Brown, & Hiestand, 1993a, 1993b). These documents prepared by three nurse historians, Nettie Birnbach, Janie Brown, and Wanda Hiestand, serve as an ethical compass for nurse historians. In this chapter, Birnbach describes the genesis of these two documents and why she and her colleagues needed to develop professional standards and guidelines. The readers find the reprint of these two important documents and can apply them to their own research.

While the reprinting of the Ethical Guidelines and Standards of Professional Conduct in the previous chapter is important, the application of such documents is essential. Chapter 13, "Using Ethical Guidelines and Standards of Professional Conduct," explores the use of these two documents. In this chapter, Lewenson and Herrmann offer points to consider when reflecting upon ethical issues that may arise when doing historical research. They present two case studies to help think through some of those points. Lewenson and Herrmann analyze the decisions made in the two cases using some of the ideas found in Birnbach, Brown, and Hiestand's *Ethical Guidelines for the Nurse Historian* and *Standards of Professional Conduct for Historical Inquiry in Nursing* (1993a, 1993b). This chapter hopes to engage the reader in an ongoing discussion about ethics and the historical research process.

Doing historical research requires time and money; however, convincing funding agencies of these needs may be even more daunting for historians in search of scarce research dollars. Nurse historians Jean C. Whelan and Cynthia Anne Connolly describe in Chapter 14, "Funding for Historical Research," the steps involved in finding funding for historical research. These two successfully funded researchers include practical advice on obtaining financial support in both the federal and private sectors. From their own experiences, they pragmatically outline how, when, where, and why historical research can be funded. This chapter could easily have been the first in this book, because without funding, there may not be historical research.

Three appendixes complete the book and add important essential information for the nurse historian. Appendix 1, "Artifacts: Additional Resources," offers an annotated list of resources that historians can access for more information about artifacts. The second and third appendies contain updated information from the files of the American Association for the History of Nursing (AAHN) Web site (http://aahn.org/). AAHN Executive Secretary and Webmaster Janet L. Fickeissen presents a listing of nursing history centers, archives, and museums in Appendix 2. In Appendix 3, Fickeissen provides an updated listing of historical resources that can be found on the Internet. These useful references will assist nurse historians, both new and seasoned, in locating support for their work. We decided to include these two appendices in the book knowing full well that many of the Internet sites will change over time. However, we still felt it was important as a starting point to include this information and encourage the reader go to the AAHN Web site (http://aahn.org/) for a more complete and updated listing of resources.

Our goal in creating *Capturing Nursing History: A Guide to Historical Methods in Research* is to further a conversation about doing historical research. This book will serve as a guide to those who are interested in doing this kind of work and will encourage thoughtful, reflective dialogue among those who do. Each of our contributors has added their insights based on the many years of experience of doing historical research. We wanted to collect their wisdom and share it with a larger audience who will find support for their work in the pages of this book.

Sandra B. Lewenson, EdD, RN, FAAN
Eleanor Krohn Herrmann, EdD, RN, FAAN

REFERENCES

Birnbach, N., Brown, J., & Hiestand, W. (1993a). Ethical guidelines for the nurse historian. *American Association for the History of Nursing Bulletin, Spring* (38), 4.

Birnbach, N., Brown, J., & Hiestand, W. (1993b). Standards of professional conduct for historical inquiry in nursing. *American Association for the History of Nursing Bulletin, Spring* (38), 5.

Buck, J. (2004). Home hospice versus home health: Cooperation, competition, and cooptation. *Nursing History Review, 12*, 25–46.

D'Antonio, P. (in press). Conceptual and methodological issues in historical research. In S. B. Lewenson & E. K. Herrmann (Eds.), *Capturing nursing history: A guide to historical methods in research*. New York: Springer Publishing.

Grypma, S. (2005). Critical issues in the use of biographic methods in nursing history. *Nursing History Review, 13*, 171–187.

Herrmann, E. K. (2006). *Turn-of-century nursing artifacts* (3rd edition—revised & expanded). Lanoka Harbor, NJ: American Association for the History of Nursing.

Acknowledgments

There comes a time in every project that you need to take a moment to reflect on all the people who have come to your aid. This book could not have been done alone, in isolation, or in any way without the countless number of people who have supported this venture.

First, we want to acknowledge historians throughout the decades who have studied nursing history. This includes all the historians who thought nursing was a worthwhile subject to examine, all the historians who are nurses and who value the historical context of our profession, all the lovers of nursing and history who read and use historical research in nursing to inform their lives, and to all the future nurse historians who will continue to explore the past.

Second, this work reflects the passion that so many of us who study nursing history share. We acknowledge the many contributors who gave their wisdom, time, and joy of history with us. We want to thank each one of them for their Herculean efforts.

Third, we want to thank our respective families for all their support throughout the writing of this book. Sandy's husband, Richard Lewenson, and their children, Jennie and Chris Hansen, and Nicole and Jeff Shargel provided much needed understanding throughout the year, cheering us on, and at times, critiquing our work. The rest of her family and friends supported us as well, like all of the Nibur clan and her sister, Michelle Kalina. Eleanor's husband, Lawrence Herrmann, a staunch supporter of nursing history, especially at the American Association for the History of Nursing auctions, provided ongoing encouragement throughout the endeavor. Thanks also to Jane Krohn Gates, Eleanor's sister who was her partner in seeking antiques, especially those related to nursing; Eleanor expresses love and gratitude for sharing those adventures. For all of our family, friends, and colleagues, we are forever grateful.

During the process of writing together, we became great friends and served as a personal cheering squad for each other throughout the process of writing. Collaboration for us became another way of capturing nursing history that has been meaningful and rewarding.

One final person who we would like to thank is Sally Barhydt at Springer Publishing who believed in the relevance of this work and gave us the opportunity to have it published. We thank everyone who has had a hand in *Capturing Nursing History: A Guide to Historical Methods in Research* and extend our heartfelt appreciation to you all.

CHAPTER ONE

Why Do Historical Research?

Sandra B. Lewenson and Eleanor Krohn Herrmann

WHY STUDY NURSING HISTORY?

During the mid-20th century, Mary M. Roberts inscribed one of the copies of her book *American Nursing: History and Interpretation* with the following wish, "May the future of nursing be even brighter than its past." The profession of nursing had passed a 50-year mark celebrating the first printing of the esteemed *American Journal of Nursing* (AJN). Roberts's book marked the anniversary of this journal as well as proposed to tell the history of nursing up until 1952 when nursing underwent dramatic changes in the organization of the profession. The AJN's board had elected Mary M. Roberts to write the story of the start of the AJN, and she was given a "free hand in designing the scope of the work" (Leone, 1954, p. v.). Roberts decided to go further than just tell the story of the founding of the AJN. Instead, she used the book as an opportunity to examine the historical development of nursing during the end of the 19th century and the first half of the 20th. The book offered "more information, deeper analysis, and a broader view of the society which nursing served and the challenges which nursing met" (Leone, 1954, p. vi). Roberts's history prompted Leone to write in the foreword of the book that "history can become our wise teacher" (p. vii).

Years later, Palmer (1976) wrote that the "major value of history, historians, and methods of historical thinking is not in their contribution of and to things past, but in the knowledge and involvement history establishes in everyday people in the everyday world" (p. 118). That understanding of history provides us with a way of knowing what happened before, a way of understanding current issues, and offers a way to glean an insight of the future.

History teaches us who we are. We, as a profession, need to understand this as history offers us an identity that we can use to help us grow and evolve. *Nursing History Review*'s first editor, Joan Lynaugh (1996), put it this way: "history is our source of identity, our cultural DNA; it affords us collective immortality" (p. 1). She goes on to say that "history yields self-knowledge by structuring a mind capable of imagining new ideas, values, and experiences, thus creating and recreating culture and discipline" (p. 1). Knowing the past allows nurses to imagine the possibilities in their day-to-day world and on into the future.

If, indeed, "history matters" as the second *Nursing History Review* editor Patricia D'Antonio (2003) stated, then the ability to capture and study history becomes a core mission of the profession. D'Antonio sees history as an "overarching conceptual framework that allows us to more fully understand the disparate meaning of nursing and the different experiences of nursing" (p. 1). Nurses learn from past experiences of other nurses, their nursing leaders, and the myriad of contextual factors that shape the past and influence present-day practice settings. By considering history as an overarching framework, nurse historians see their role as essential to the health and well-being of the profession itself. Historical research enables nurses to explore their past and thus become critically aware of their professional identity and meaning. Yet, to want to study nursing history, one needs to recognize the value of history and then learn the tools by which to study it.

It has been said many times and in many ways that nursing history is important, relevant, and futuristic. Few, however, discuss how one learns nursing history and how one becomes a nurse historian. Rafferty (1997/1998) speaks to this by saying that one becomes a historian by doing historical research. This chapter examines the why and how of becoming a nurse historian. Within this first chapter, Herrmann and Lewenson reflect upon what prompted them and others to seek this type of research trajectory. Who the historian is and what their ideas and values are have an impact on the kind of research trajectory they select and the subsequent outcomes they find (Rafferty, 1997/1998). Equally important are the reasons why one studies nursing history written by others, who the historian is, and how to engage others to recognize, value, and study nursing history.

BECOMING A NURSE HISTORIAN

Little is known about the reasons for becoming a nurse historian and why this might be important to historical research. Herrmann (2002) wrote that "until the stories are teased out and told in their fullest, information about the incipient stages of becoming a nurse historian are often overlooked, not recognized, or not given credit for their impact" (p. 1). How we learn about nursing history and how we become nurse historians is important to understand and to share with others. What triggers our interest and "professional metamorphoses" in becoming nurse historians may be as simple as "... travel, chance meetings or introductions and happenstance" (p. 1). For example, historian Carol Daisy (1991) began her journey by exploring the professional life of Annie Goodrich after buying Goodrich's nursing pin in an antique shop. The noted nurse historian Josephine Dolan expressed an early "distaste" for nursing history based upon the boring course she sat through while in nursing school. However, she became a devout lifelong nurse historian after hearing how the then dean of the University of Connecticut School of Nursing spoke of, "her grandfather, a clerical missionary in Turkey, who helped Florence Nightingale at the Barrack Hospital in Scutari during the Crimean War by setting up a bakery and establishing a laundry to wash the soldiers' clothing" (Herrmann, 2002, p. 1).

For others, such as the former American Association for the History of Nursing (AAHN) president Nettie Birnbach, her interest in nursing history started with her love for reading. Herrmann (2002) describes Birnbach as an "avid reader" who was inspired early on by biographies of Madame Curie, Ignaz Semmelweis, and Walter Reed. Later Birnbach's interests expanded to include courses in history, among them courses on the American Civil War and Irish history. Birnbach's doctoral dissertation that addressed the evolution of nurse licensure began her work in historical research in nursing. Herrmann (2002) describes how others in nursing, such as *Nursing History Review* editor Patricia D'Antonio, began college as a history major and eventually switched to nursing. While attending the University of Virginia where history of nursing is valued, D'Antonio successfully merged her two interests, that of nursing and history. For historian Joy Buck, family trips to the cemeteries where their family ancestors were buried triggered an early interest in nursing history.

The noted nursing educator Isabel Stewart's interest in nursing history, which later led to the publication of *A Short History of Nursing* in 1920, was spurred on by her curiosity to "know what made people do things that they did" (Flack, 1927, p. 555). This interest in history continued as Stewart proceeded through nursing school at Johns Hopkins. Stewart recognized that history influenced the growth of nursing at Johns Hopkins, and she sought to learn more about these influences through historical research. Stewart influenced her students at Teacher's College to pursue historical study in nursing's history. Holly Flack, a student of Stewart's at Columbia's Teacher's College and elected vice-president of the then newly formed History-of-Nursing Society at Teacher's College, was one of the students Stewart inspired to organize the History-of-Nursing Society. Flack and her classmates met with Stewart's colleague and predecessor Adelaide Nutting to ask for her input into the formation of this society. Flack wrote that Nutting supported this venture and agreed to serve as the History-of-Nursing Society's Honorary President. Stewart agreed to act as the Faculty Advisor. Both nursing leaders encouraged and supported the founding of the History-of-Nursing Society. Flack wrote the following account of her experience:

> Miss Nutting was determined that future nurses should have an opportunity to know the background of their professional life. Lavinia L. Dock, who was at that time secretary of the International Council of Nurses, and a profound student, joined her in her search for all available historical data.... It was the conviction of the worth-whileness of this material that led these indefatigable women to carry out so stupendous an undertaking, involving as it did many long evenings at the end of busy days of hospital routine. (Flack, 1927, p. 555)

Understanding what triggered an interest in historical research and how one becomes a nurse historian may help to encourage future nurses to select this research trajectory. If nursing history is important and matters, then we need historians to study it. We need to be able to support the growth and development of this type of researcher. Telling the stories about how we became interested in nursing history and how we learned the research methodology supports this effort. In the next section, the authors of this book share their own stories about becoming nurse historians. Through this self-reflective exercise, we hope to encourage others to reflect and value their own development as historians and to encourage others on their way of becoming one.

Eleanor Krohn Herrmann's Story

My interest in history began at an early age and gradually evolved over time. Without initially recognizing it, I was becoming the family historian because I repeatedly wanted to hear the stories about my Swedish heritage. That curiosity and sense of continuity spilled over into other areas and created the "benchmarks" for me. For example, as a youngster I wondered who had built and lived in our family home that had the inscription, "R. Fuller—1832," chiseled into the stone of the front doorstep. I was not yet a historian and had no training in historical research, but an elementary exploration of town and church records yielded some of the answers I sought. I gave the results of that investigation to my mother as a Christmas gift. Another experience in my early life furthered my growing passion for uncovering history. My best friend and I decided that we should ride our bicycles over what we believed must have been the route that Daniel Shays took when leading an armed uprising to protest high taxation in Massachusetts (1786–1787). We pedaled our way in the summer heat between Sheffield and Great Barrington. That exploration into Shays's journey now seems to have been a harbinger of what was to become my personal and serious journey into the study of nursing history later in my life.

As a nursing major in college, another benchmark incidence occurred. While studying pharmacology we learned how the discovery of penicillin had dramatically changed health care. It was then that I made the connection between science and the history of nursing that I had witnessed when a family member, years before, had been treated with mustard plasters for what was then called double pneumonia. The significance of that revelation remained with me throughout my nursing career as an educator. Every class I taught included the background of the subject I was presenting. Sometimes it was in the form of words, other times with the inclusion of artifacts, but I simply could not omit the inclusion of nursing history. Without it, it was like starting to read a book in the middle.

An opportunity to work in Belize, Central America, led to another benchmark. After months of working on a curriculum revision, I suggested that we include a history of the school in the final document. My Belizean colleagues and I wrote that history using stories about what they had experienced. I realized then that I wanted and needed to learn more about the historical research method. After returning to New York City, I was encouraged by Eleanor Lambertsen, the Dean of the Cornell University School of Nursing, to enroll in doctoral study at Teacher's College, Columbia University. When it was time to select a topic for my dissertation, I decided to research the history of Belizean nursing education. That led to taking courses in history and historical methodology and having the good fortune of having the esteemed nurse historian, M. Louise Fitzpatrick, as my mentor. An outcome of the final research was the publication of the dissertation, the first book about Belizean nursing that had ever been published (Herrmann, 1985). It was cited by the Pan American Health Organization, the Latin American arm of the World Health Organization, as an example for other developing countries that wanted to record their history of nursing.

Sandra B. Lewenson's Story

I decided to complete my doctorate at Teacher's College, Columbia University in New York City because I fell in love with the history of nursing that seemed to live in every nook and cranny of the college. Further, the questions I raised about the value of nursing and the loss of our historical memory about past political activity of nurses also seemed to fit the historical method, which was an acceptable research design at Teacher's College. Yet, I was a novice in nursing history, only recently engaged in the academic pursuit of knowledge about nursing's past and what it meant to contemporary nursing. I was also a novice at using the historical method. Consequently, my doctoral course work led me to courses such as the history of education in America and historical design. To extend my knowledge, I joined the now-defunct Society for Nursing History at Teacher's College and the newly formed American Association for the History of Nursing.

As I developed my dissertation questions, I found myself on unsteady ground, faced with issues that all historians are faced with. The topic I selected was too broad, and there was a question about the adequacy of data. I decided to approach my topic by designing a study that examined the records of the four nursing organizations that had formed between 1873 and 1920. I explored whether nurses, through their professional organizations, supported the efforts of late 19th- and early 20th-century women to obtain the right to vote. While my primary sources provided useful data, I needed to be comfortable with the ambiguity and conflicting stories that I also found in the data. This comfort with ambiguity, which Lynaugh and Reverby (1987) identified as part of the historian's dilemma, meant that I would never know the facts entirely. As a historian, I could only piece together a part of the "story" using the data that I uncovered. Becoming a historian means being able to accept this inadequacy of data and to continually look to find data that would support a better understanding of the subject under study.

I finished my doctoral work in 1989; I spent the rest of my career extending my knowledge about nursing history and historiography and applying it to my work in nursing education and nursing research. The people I turned to for this knowledge have been the nurse historians and historians of nursing that make up a small cadre of outstanding researchers interested in making sense of our current health care environment. Nurses who are historians and historians who study nursing provide the historical antecedents for questions raised today as well as shape the historical method that is used.

ENGAGING OTHERS

What many nurse historians have in common is a curiosity for learning and the need to seek out meaning about the world around them. Whether through reading, exploring, traveling, or thinking, historians evolve, like Herrmann said, over time. Part of mentoring the next generation of historical researchers in nursing begins in nursing education programs. Including discussions about nursing history in nursing education requires several skills.

First, faculty need to value nursing history and want to include it within the nursing curriculum. Either through a separate history of nursing course, or integrated within the curriculum, faculty need to make a place for it so that students can learn to appreciate the profession's history, use historical evidence in practice, and perhaps become historical researchers in the future. Keeling (2001), author of the American Association for the History of Nursing's Position Paper on Integrating History in the Curriculum, stated that by including nursing history in the curriculum, we will be able to

> educate rather than "train" our students. In so doing, we will give them a sense of professional identity, a useful methodological research skill, and a context for evaluating information. Overall, it will provide students with the cognitive flexibility that will be required for the formation and navigation of tomorrow's health care environment.

Second, faculty need to know what and how to teach history. Too often history is omitted in classroom or clinical content because the faculty does not know the history or there is too much other material to cover (Lewenson, 2004). History needs to be taught in an interesting and creative manner that stokes the fires of creativity, inquisitiveness, and exploration in others. Too often we remember our own boring course in nursing history, or more too often, we remember nothing or very little instruction about nursing's history. As mentioned earlier in this chapter, Josephine Dolan's love of history was rekindled by her teacher's presentation of her own family background and her father's relationship with Florence Nightingale. Yet, according to Herrmann (2002), Dolan's initial response to nursing history had been a "boring" course in history and only after hearing the excitement presented by another teacher did she become excited by the past.

In 1929, Eppley, an early nursing educator, emphasized the need to creatively present nursing history in class. She did this through a vignette where one nursing student asks a fellow nursing student, Brownie, where she was going. Upon hearing Brownie's answer she replied, "Oh, yes, you will have a wonderful time while I must go to that old history of nursing class. I do not see any value in spending our time hearing about some old woman who lived years and years ago" (Eppley, 1929, p. 1322). Eppley said that faculty needed to know history as well as to "enjoy reading it, talking it, [and] searching for facts" (p. 1322).

Third, faculty need to rely on historical research for the evidence they can use in teaching and in practice. Historiography, such as Keeling's (2006) study about the autonomous practice of visiting nurses at the Henry Street Settlement on the Lower East Side of New York City in the late 19th and early 20th centuries, provides historical evidence that contributes to better understanding of some of the professional boundary–related issues faced by contemporary nurses. The historical evidence adds depth to current discussions concerning such issues as prescriptive privileges for nurse practitioners, autonomy of practice, or the move toward the Doctor of Nursing Practice. Buck's (2007) examination of the transitions in care following the start of the American hospice movement causes nurses to critically think about their ideas about death and dying. The idea that good nursing care was the basis for care of the dying patient is played out in the historical research and lends itself to opening a broader discussion for nurses today. Without historical analysis of the data, we would miss the nuances and meaning behind much of the work we do in nursing today. Understanding the relevance of historical research and using this research in teaching and practice lends itself to perpetuating the idea of valuing and using historical research design.

Fourth, faculty need to see the value in historical research design. Too often we hear concerns that doctoral committees and university tenure committees alike discourage historiography as a research design, thus making it more difficult for nurse historians to be granted tenure and promotion. Students with an interest in history are often dissuaded from pursuing that type of research. Along the same lines, with little federal grant money available, historical research is only rarely funded, thus detracting academicians from pursuing historical designs in research. Historical research provides us with essential, thought-provoking analysis that we need to evolve as a profession.

Finally, faculty need to impart the value of historical research design for students to pursue this course of study in the future. Given the perceived lack of support and value of historical research, it takes a Herculean effort to encourage and mentor the work of those interested in pursuing historical research designs. In 1927 students in Isabel Stewart's history course at Teacher's College were so excited by Stewart's "dynamic enthusiasm" they organized a History-of-Nursing Society (Flack, 1927, p. 553). The purpose of the new society was:

1. To provide a medium for bringing together students and others who are deeply interested in the serious study of nursing history including international nursing relationships.

2. To foster methods of historical study and to encourage the preparation and publication of reliable articles and reports dealing with nursing history.
3. To collect and preserve historical materials related to nursing, including anything on hospitals, public health, etc., which is likely to be a direct and vital interest to the student of nursing history now or in the future.
4. To honor pioneers and leaders who have made some substantial contribution to nursing history and to cultivate and maintain cordial relationships with representatives of nursing in our own and other countries.
5. To keep in close touch with current developments in nursing, both national and international, and to cultivate the long view and the broad view in dealing with modern problems in nursing. (Flack, 1927, p. 554)

Faculty like Stewart and the many that have come after her inspire students with their insight, interpretation, and enthusiasm for history. At the American Association for the History of Nursing annual meetings, doctoral students often accompany their faculty to these meetings. The faculty/student groups present their research, support each other at their presentations, and encourage continued interest in historical research. The doctoral luncheon discussions held at the annual meetings are well attended by doctoral students and stimulate thoughtful interchanges and reveal evolving studies. Mentorship by faculty provides the impetus to develop nurse historians and thus has the potential to exponentially foster historical knowledge building.

CAPTURING NURSING HISTORY

This first chapter in *Capturing Nursing History: A Guide to Historical Methods in Research* is meant to encourage us to look at why we become nurse historians and how we can develop others to recognize the relevance of historical research. The historical method requires interest in the subject, creativity in organizing the data, and comfort with the vagaries presented by this methodology. This chapter frames the remainder of the chapters, explaining why one becomes a nurse historian, how to engage others in this research process, and how to support the study of nursing history.

The book serves as a collection of ideas about doing historiography written from the standpoint of different nurse historians and not typically found in other written discussions on this subject. Each historian brings to the work their own personal reasons for selecting this type of research design. They also bring to light their own experiences and share them with the reader. When we explore how to capture nursing's history, it requires us to look at various ways in which this can be done and various ways in which we interpret the history. Each historian approaches the process from their own perspective, thus adding to the larger picture. The various brush strokes of each historian, like a painter, build on each other to provide a more coherent understanding of how to do historical research and why we do historical research. Each of the contributors in this text, like the artist, adds to the broader discussion about capturing nursing's history using historiography as a way to provide that insight.

REFERENCES

Buck, J. (2007). Reweaving a tapestry of care. *Nursing History Review, 15,* 113–145.

Daisy, C. A. (1991). Historiography: Searching for Annie Goodrich. *Western Journal of Nursing Research, 13*(3), 409–413.

D'Antonio, P. (2003). Editor's note. *Nursing History Review, 11,* 1.

Eppley, C. E. (1929). Teaching history of nursing. *American Journal of Nursing, 29*(11), 1322.

Flack, H. (1927). A history-of-nursing society: Organized by nursing students of Teachers College. *American Journal of Nursing, 27*(7), 553–555.

Herrmann, E. (1985). *Origins of tomorrow: A history of Belizean nursing education.* Belize: Ministry of Health.

Herrmann, E. (2002). Message from the president: Lessons from our own stories. *American Association for the History of Nursing Bulletin, 73,* 1–2.

Leone, L. P. (1954). Foreword. In M. M. Roberts (Ed.), *American nursing: History and interpretation* (pp. v–vii). New York: Macmillan Company.

Lewenson, S. B. (2004). Integrating nursing history in the curriculum. *Journal of Professional Nursing, 20*(6), 374–380.

Lynaugh, J. E. (1996). Editorial. *Nursing History Review, 4,* 1.

Lynaugh, J., & Reverby, S. (1987). Thoughts on the nature of history. *Nursing Research, 36*(1), 4, 69.

Keeling, A. (2001). *Nursing history in the curriculum: Preparing nurses for the 21st century.* AAHN position paper. Retrieved May 7, 2007, from http://aahn.org/position.htm

Keeling, A. (2006). Medicines in the work of Henry Street Settlement Visiting Nurses. *Nursing History Review, 14,* 7–30.

Palmer, I. S. (1976). The role of history in the preparation of nurse leadership. *Nursing Forum, 15*(2), 116–122.

Rafferty, A. M. (1997/1998). Researching nursing's history: Writing, researching and reflexivity in nursing history. *Nurse Researcher, 5*(2), 5–16.

CHAPTER TWO

Conceptual and Methodological Issues in Historical Research

Patricia D'Antonio

At a 1994 research conference, the distinguished historian John Lewis Gaddis (2002) asked the eminent historian William H. McNeil to explain historical research methods to a group of social, physical, and biological scientists. McNeil described his approach:

> I get curious about a problem and start reading up on it. What I read causes me to redefine the problem. Redefining the problem causes me to shift the direction of what I'm reading. That in turn further reshapes the problem, which further redirects the reading. I go back and forth like this until it feels right, then I write it up and ship it off to a publisher. (Gaddis, 2002, p. 48)

Experienced scholars will recognize two essential truths in McNeil's description. First, it rather accurately describes the very real (and very messy) process of scientific reasoning that occurs before any finding, in any discipline, finds its way into the neat categories of *problem, methods, data,* and *analysis* that appear in most scholarly journals. Second, McNeil's description just as accurately captures

This chapter originated in 2005 as an editorial in the *Nursing History Review* (13), 1–3. Sections reprinted with permission of Springer Publishing Company. Acknowledgments: I am grateful to the participants in the History and Health Care Seminar at the Barbara Bates Center for the Study of the History of Nursing for their valuable comments and suggestions.

the peculiar inexactness with which historians define, delineate, and defend their particular research methodology. A compelling body of literature exists that describes specialized technical procedures for evaluating historical documents, interpreting oral history data, and statistically managing large blocks of data. But only a very small number address the overarching question: How do historians actually do historical research?

It must be noted that this lack of methodological self-reflexivity has not interfered with the construction of sophisticated historical studies in nursing. The past 25 years, in fact, represent something of a renaissance of nursing history both in the United States and around the world. As I have argued elsewhere, historical research about the work and worth of nurses has reshaped scholars' and clinicians' sense of the historical hospital, the birth of babies, and the role of women in their families and their communities (D'Antonio, 1999). Still, as Gaddis (2002) points out, methodological innocence, or the reluctance to directly engage how we do historical research, leads to methodological vulnerability (p. 51). Not being able to explain how we do what we do leads to a diminished recognition of the specialized skills necessary for this research discipline; to an unfounded reliance on the seemingly scientific processes of document validity and reliability that have little connection to historians' actual work; and, perhaps most significantly, to an inability to coherently teach historical reasoning as the foundation of clinical practice and humanistic understanding.

This chapter, then, lays out what I believe to be key conceptual and methodological issues that might begin to address the question: How do historians actually do historical research? I offer five key conceptual issues. Four of these issues—the interconnectedness of variables or concepts, the manipulation of such variables or concepts in time and place, contextualization, and judgment—borrow heavily from Gaddis's (2002) formulation; and the final conceptual issue—a tolerance for ambiguity—draws from other perspectives. These conceptual issues capture the particular strength and uniqueness of historical research. They might also, I hope, provide a way to more concretely structure the dreaded methods and data analysis section of grant applications and manuscripts intended for clinical journals. Rather than, for example, vaguely referencing the "methods of social history" (and hoping, as I have many times, that no one will notice that social history is a framework and not a method!), one might speak more specifically about the questions that will be raised, the data that will be analyzed, the variables or concepts of interest, how such variables of concepts will be positioned both in place and over time, the specifics of context, and the issue upon which a judgment (or an assessment) will be brought to bear. This chapter also suggests three methodological issues—reading, representation, and writing—with which historians grapple. I speak deliberately of *methodological issues* rather than *methods*. Historical research is a disciplined mode of inquiry, but it is not inherently rule- or procedure-based (although some of the particular methods of history, such as oral history or microhistory, may have their suggestions about how best to proceed and the issues to consider). I will also add that these methodological issues are by no means unique to historical research; they represent historians' shared commitment to the wonderful enterprise of knowledge development for the profession (D'Antonio, 2006). But these methodological issues do assume a somewhat different form when historians call them into play. In the end, they remind us that our unique methodological tool is time and, as Gaddis so eloquently states, we historians use the distance of time to lift us above the familiar to experience vicariously what we cannot experience directly: a broader view (p. 5).

CONCEPTUAL ISSUES

As Gaddis (2002) argues, four conceptual, or what he describes as procedural, commitments underpin historical methodology and differentiate this particular methodology from the positivist principles that underpin other scientific pursuits.

Interconnectedness of Variables

First, historians hold steadfast to the belief that all variables are intrinsically interconnected. Rather than wonder which is likely to produce the largest magnitude of change, historians wonder how variables interact within time and place to effect change. Consider, for example, Joy Buck's (2007) analysis of the trans-Atlantic hospice movement and its success in changing the culture of dying in the later decades of the 20th century. Buck brings together such variables as charismatic leadership, personal experiences, shifting professional paradigms, and strong faith traditions. She then places such variables within a particular time in which a growing public discourse about the quality of living and dying opened a particular place for experimentation with both forms of care and the clinical roles of nursing and medicine. Buck does not privilege any one variable over another. Rather, the strength of her analysis lies in her explication of the intimate connectedness of relationships, the religious exemplars, and some nurses' search for new sources of power and authority that eventually created a specialized and, as importantly, reimbursable model of care for the terminally ill.

Manipulation of Variables

How, though, do historians judge which variables are important? Historians, Gaddis (2002) explains, conduct "experiments of the mind." They mentally manipulate the effects of variables within their time and place to judge relative significances. Julie Fairman (1999), in her analysis of physicians, nurse practitioners, and the process of clinical thinking, conducts one such experiment. Rather than approach the experiences of physicians and nurses in the 1960s through a traditional medical history framework, Fairman deliberately (and explicitly) wonders what that history might look like if told from the perspective of nurse practitioners. Her "experiment of the mind," then, is to use the nurse practitioner movement as the central position from which to view both the actual work of the health care system and the intellectual framing of knowledge domains. This experiment proved fruitful. Fairman ultimately argued that factors (or, to return to our particular conceptualizing, *variables*) such as changes in nursing and medical education and practice, federal entitlement policies, and economics supported changes in nurse practitioner knowledge and skill domains through a process of negotiation rather than delegation. This, she pointed out, is a critically important distinction: Physician and nurse practitioner negotiations involve mutual power and choice and were not the one-sided process implied by delegated duties.

Contextualization and Causation

Third, historians emphasize contextual specificity. In Gaddis's (2002) words, they select a certain event, place it within its time, and then work backwards in time assigning, in the process, more importance to immediate rather than remote causes of the event (p. 34). That is, historians seek to place their event (or person, or concept, or institution) of interest in a particular place at a particular moment, not to provide the obligatory "immigration, industrialization, and urbanization" paragraph I might inadvertently—and incorrectly—use when discussing 19th-century American nursing. But rather, we do so to explicate causality—to demonstrate some relationship of dependency that moves our understanding of an event from a simple description of what happened to an explanation and understanding of *why* it happened. And, Gaddis and others remind us, when considering the dimensions of this relationship of dependency, and when assessing the relative importance of the variables that form this relationship, more weight must go to those contextual factors nearer in time and place to the event of interest (Howell & Prevenier, 2001, p. 128).

Arlene Keeling's (2004) work on critical care nursing illustrates the precision of this process. Her historical event, so to speak, was the inception and proliferation of cardiac care units in the 1960s and, in particular, the place of nursing within this critically important development. She identifies the first such units at Bethany Hospital in Kansas City and Presbyterian Hospital in Philadelphia, and, in particular, the importance of the relationship between the physician, Laurence Meltzer, and the nurse, Rose Pinneo. Keeling, in her published manuscript, draws the reader into her arguments about cardiac care units and the blurring of boundaries between medicine and nursing by moving from broad to narrow contextual issues. But the contextual factors at play in her arguments about causality actually begin with—and have more data associated with and thus more weight assigned to—the immediately pressing issues in the nursing care of patients with myocardial infarction. With that established, she then moves outward to the other contextual pieces within this relationship: to new technological and scientific advances in cardiology, to the possibilities of space-age technologies, and, finally, to the broadest contextual issue—still critically important but less immediately vexing to Meltzer and Pinneo's treatment of patients with potentially fatal arrhythmias—of the "coronary problem" of post-war America.

Judgments

Fourth, in Gaddis's formulation, historians make judgments. They make, in the end, some kind of statement about where the variable, object, event, or actor of interest lies along the spectrum that runs from the admirable to the abominable. In a similar way, Paul Forman (1991) argues that the hallmark characteristic of history's intellectual independence is its reciprocal responsibility to critically and forthrightly assess meaning and significance. Such statements need to be direct. They might follow the example of Margarete Sandelowski (2000) who, in her work on nursing and technology, is quite clear in her assessment of the ambiguity in and the problematic nature of that historical relationship. Nurses did play a central role in the technological transformation of medical practice and hospital care, she argues, but nursing gave more to technology than technology ever gave to nursing. In her work, technology never redefined the status of nurses in the way it did that of physicians. Indeed, she concludes—never mincing her words—although nurses certainly "acquired new knowledge and skill, what nurses gained most of all was new (and, arguably, more) work to do" (p. 28).

Ambiguity

Finally, I would suggest that historians have a tolerance, and perhaps even a preference, for ambiguity and uncertainty. They prefer to "complicate" (one of my favorite buzzwords) that which seems self-evident and to concentrate on the rather complicated space where ideas about people, events, or issues collide with the reality of personalities, politics, or day-to-day practice. Geertje Boschma's (1999) work on mental health nursing in Dutch asylums in the late 19th and early 20th centuries might stand as one such example. Psychiatrists in Dutch asylums, she points out, like their counterparts in other Western countries, embraced new somatic therapies and a system of mental health nursing education. But Boschma moves beneath the official pronouncements and seemingly self-evident appearances and uncovers what she describes as inherent contradictions of which even contemporary clinicians were unaware. Most notably, Boschma points out, Dutch psychiatrists consistently emphasized nurses' new forms of training, new uniforms, and new living arrangements—using them to symbolize a more progressive and professional outlook. But in the crucible of actual practice, these attempts at modernization created as many problems as they solved. Because, she argues, such innovations were not based on any developed system of care for the mentally ill, they only turned the rhetoric of professionalization toward another way of controlling their patients' more unacceptable behaviors. I would also suggest that historians' tolerance and preference for ambiguity accounts for the fact that, search as one might, it is almost impossible to find that sentence or paragraph that will tell our more quantitatively oriented colleagues exactly what it is we are going to do or have done in our historical studies. Historians adore discussing the permutations of, for example, social feminism, cultural feminism, second wave feminism, and so on and so forth, without ever pausing to wonder—and indeed such a pause would seem beside the point—if there existed any way to operationalize the definition of feminism itself. My own search for a precise definition of social history for this chapter turned up only Sigurður Gylfi Magnússon's (2003) assertion that one need not delve into attempts to explain the framework social history (and, parenthetically, his intent was to discuss the method of microhistory) because "most people in the field have a pretty clear idea of what social history is all about" (p. 702). Yikes! But fortunately, Magnússon did suggest that most social historians might agree with Jürgen Kocka's (1996, 2003) definition, which I offer and will use if pressed. Social history, then, is a "subfield of historical studies which deals mainly with social structures, processes and experiences, for example..."—and now one would choose among—"...classes and strata, ethnic and religious groups, migrations and families, business structures and entrepreneurship, mobility, gender relations, urbanization, or patterns of rural life" (as cited in Magnússon, 2003, p. 702). We can easily add our own as well: race and race relations, or perhaps geography and place. And then move to what we really want to do as we move into methodological issues.

METHODOLOGICAL ISSUES

It has become something of a truism to state that all historical research begins with a question. In fact, the meaning of history to a practice profession such as nursing lies in our questions: questions that are quite different than those raised by other methods; and questions that may escape notice in the press of daily practice (D'Antonio, 2006). But not all questions are historical questions. And not all legitimate historical questions lead inevitably to a research project. As McNeil's confession at the beginning of this chapter reveals, the movement from historical interest to question to research begins with and continues throughout the process of reading.

Reading

Reading as a methodological tool has received almost no attention. Trained historians, reading since their undergraduate days, simply assume its place in their methodological armentarium and see no need to expound upon it although it forms the basis for some important tools of the historian's trade—the published book reviews and historiographic essays that are an important part of the advancement of historical knowledge. And much of the methodological steps in reading remain constant across disciplines. One reads, of course, to discover what is known, what is contested, and what remains to be discovered about the event, object, person, concept, or moment in time of interest. Thus, one reads—and writes about—historical studies much as one does in any other discipline. Catherine Choy (2003) presents a cogent synthesis of such reading in her introduction to *Empire of Care*—a synthesis that might be alternatively termed a "state of the science" essay in another research field. By drawing on a wide body of research in Asian American migration, labor, and women's histories, Choy ultimately develops a new and compelling rationale for approaching the historical experiences of Filipino nurses in the United States, not just as fellow professionals but also as a window into the global and colonial dimensions of a predominately female migrant work flow.

One also reads history to place one's event, object, person, concept, or moment in time within a particular framework of historical inquiry. Over the past 20 years, most histories of nursing have been placed within the framework of social history. The fit between nursing and social history is quite good. Social history's emphasis on uncovering and understanding the experiences of those who had been heretofore invisible in the formal historical record does work well for those who would uncover the experiences of nurses who might be considered as invisible in health and home care systems. Particular subfields within social history, such as women's history, labor history, and African American history, have also influenced historical studies in nursing, as have other fields of historical inquiry. Intellectual history, institutional history, political history, to name but a few, have all emerged as fields whose historical perspectives help shed light on events, objects, persons, and concepts that have been of interest to researchers in nursing.

Why might one narrow one's frame of understanding a historical event, person, or concept by placing it within a particular field of inquiry? Such placement brings methodological discipline and coherency to the processes of reading, researching, representation, and writing. Early in the research process, it structures the formulation of the initial historical questions that will guide subsequent research. Later in the research process, it guides how one decides not only what data is needed but also, and perhaps most importantly, the relative significance of identified data. And finally, such placement directs the particular generalizations that might be drawn from one's study and the judgments that one might make about meaning, identity, worth, or work. Consider, for example, Margaret Shkimba and Karen Flynn's (2005) analysis of the experiences of young black Caribbean and white British women who trained as nurses in the United Kingdom and then immigrated to Canada in the late 20th century. Their frames of identity theory, racialized discourses, and migration studies shaped the particular oral history questions they asked these nurses when trying to capture their perceptions of their training and the strategies they used to cope with their new countries and work environments. Data from these oral histories pointed to, as the literature they had read suggested it would, significant differences in the experiences of young black Caribbean and white British nurses. But these researchers' knowledge of the relevant historical literature also brought unexpected similarities into sharp relief. As Shkimba and Flynn conclude, these women's common identity as nurses—especially as British-trained nurses—medicated their experiences of racial and cultural disunity in Britain for the Caribbean nurses, and in Canada for both the Caribbean and the British nurses. Two additional points also bear mentioning. First, one brings the same critiques to the reading of historical literature as one brings to the sources of one's data. One must consider a book or article's purpose, the author's background and biases (or points of view), and the sources upon which an argument is built. Who an author is can sometimes be as important as what an author argues; and most of us teach our students that they need information about the author and his or her conceptual background and intellectual debts. Susan Reverby's (1989) *Ordered to Care,* for example, draws as much from her data as it does from her own experience as a labor activist and her training in labor and women's history.

Second, one reads to learn methods—to learn how to organize data, structure arguments, address significance, and draw conclusions. Emily Abel's (1994) article on family caregiving in the 19th century, for example, provides one such template that I have always found useful when writing for an academic audience. Abel begins with a story that draws her reader into her study, explains how this story fits with other historical studies, considers the strengths and weaknesses of her data, and sets up her argument about a fundamental aspect of human existence. She then lays out her data, slowly building to her conclusion. Abel cautions her reader against generalizing from a single case study—but then, in a way that is another too often unacknowledged strength of historical methodology (and another way our method is different from other, more cautious approaches), proceeds to do so anyway. Caregiving, she argues, is embedded in relationships and cannot be considered apart from them—and apart from both the emotional closeness and the tensions that can support as well as impede the delivery of family-based care.

Representation

But we do not and should not write just for academic colleagues. We, as historians, have an equally compelling responsibility to share our particular understanding of health and illnesses, people and institutions, problems and possibilities with our clinical colleagues, our students, and, perhaps most importantly, our patients and public. These audiences are, in all likelihood, less likely to be impressed with a virtuoso explication of the state of the science, historiographical significance, or methodological inventiveness. They want—and deserve—a story: a well-constructed and engaging historical narrative that deepens their understanding of resonant issues, or that raises ones that they never thought to consider. Eleanor Crowder's (2006) history of the last 50 years of the School of Nursing at the Hospital of the University of Pennsylvania, for example, is deeply informed by conceptual and methodological work on gender and its expression in women's education and types of service. But her final narrative form—written for a broader audience that includes the school's alumni—concentrates on the story itself. Her work illustrates that which binds good history to all its many audiences: a commitment to a valid interpretation of data that creates a meaningful representation of the event, person, institution, or idea under question. To paraphrase Edward Hallett Carr's (1961) famous phrase, Crowder does not assume the facts (or the data) speak for themselves. Rather, her careful crafting of a particular narrative from data in school records, annual reports, and hospital data builds upon, rather than overtly demonstrates, her expertise and decisions about what needs emphasis when. Crowder's work illustrates how, now in Carr's own words, "the facts speak only when the historian calls on them: it is he (or she) who decides to which facts to give the floor, and in what order or context" (p. 9).

In many respects, this process of representation—that of moving from data (or what the sources record) to interpretations (or what the sources mean)—is no different than that used by our quantitative colleagues as they move between their "data" and "analyses" sections. The raw results of a multivariate analysis might be intrinsically interesting, but they have limited usefulness until placed within a framework that explicitly explains their strengths and weaknesses and points to their particular significance. In the same way, the data that forms the basis of historical interpretations makes for wonderful reading. But they do not become historical scholarship—they do not become meaningful knowledge—until considered, critiqued, and contextualized in time and place. Historians do have a particular charge to approach this fundamental process of turning data into knowledge—that which is at the core of our research commitment—very carefully. Howell and Prevenier (2001) write that our task is to "construct interpretations responsibly, with care, and with a high degree of self-consciousness about our disabilities and the disabilities of our sources" (p. 148). I might add that applies to all researchers in all disciplines.

Historians also share with other researchers in other disciplines an active engagement in the processes of theorizing—of generating and testing broader ideas about meaning and significance that might ultimately change our perception of the work and worth of nursing. Helen Sweet (2004) and Anne Marie Rafferty and Diana Solano (2007), in their separate and collaborative work, do so when they draw on post-colonial theorizing in their analyses of British nursing. While the precise definition of "post-colonialism" remains debated, it, in general, takes as its subject the reciprocal interactions between and among Western nations and the societies they colonized in the 20th century and then analyzes source data within a model that allows for critiques of the dominance of Eurocentrism. Sweet's and Rafferty and Solano's works have been important in helping us understand the implications of nursing's power and authority—concepts that actually remain understudied and undertheorized aspects of nursing's commitment to cultural competence in global research and practice. But this historical work does have an ideological as well as theoretical and interpretative dimension.

This is not necessarily problematic. I, in fact, think some of us should engage in more explicit theorizing in our own historical work and include more perspectives from the humanities and social sciences. This process, I believe, would help us as historians continue to participate in our discipline's quest to think more deliberately about our place both in local practice and in the global mission of addressing fundamental human and social needs. But with that opportunity does come another responsibility to our data and our audience. If we choose to work within the admittedly subtle interplay between theory and ideology, we must heed the advice of, again, Howell and Prevenier (2001). "If we understand or at least acknowledge our ideological position," they write, "we can also write histories that self-consciously display those limitations to our readers. We can thus implicate our audiences in the histories we write, making them see how we see as well as what we see" (p. 148).

Writing

There are two quotations I turn to after an hour of staring at a blank page, trying to think about how my variables are interconnected, how I might manipulate them, how I might locate their contextual specificity, and what in the world I might say about the earth-shattering significance of their meaning. My first quotation provides comfort and reassurance. Trying to write history, Peter Novick once wrote, is like trying "to nail jelly to a wall" (as cited in Storey Kelleher, 2004, p. 61). The goal is a seamless and coherent argument and the end result seems innately intuitive, but the process is fraught with almost endless choices and decisions about what to include or exclude, which points in the chronology deserve more or less attention, and will anyone even care.

The second quotation, from Samuel Eliot Morison, is more bracing, as might be expected from a Boston Brahmin, an eminent Harvard history professor, and Rear Admiral in the United States Navy Reserves (Wikipedia, 2007). "First and foremost," Morison wrote—and adding the italics in case his readers missed the point, "*get writing*" (as cited in Storey Kelleher, 2004, p. 61). The point being for many, including myself: it is the very process of writing that forces one to think and rethink about the nature of one's sources, the meaning of one's variables and context, and the validity of one's interpretations. It is in this light that Nigel King (2006) explicitly presents writing as a continuation of the interpretive process. "The process of accounting for your analysis to your readers," he writes, "deepens your understanding of your data."

But, in the end, writing history is essentially a process of constructing an argument from data. It is, in David Hackett Fischer's (1970) words, constructing a "reasoned argument" that not only asserts the meaning of an event, person, institution, or idea, but provides the data that demonstrates why a reader should agree (p. 40). Consider Rose Holz's (2005) claim that nurse Adele Gordon, who owned and operated a Milwaukee birth control clinic in the 1930s, was an "impressive woman." The data in support is equally impressive: Gordon trained at the Illinois Training

School, began preliminary medical studies at the University of Chicago when female physicians were still an almost invisible minority, received several public health nursing scholarships, and earned the public admiration of at least one nationally renowned physician. And consider her argument that Gordon's clinic was more than just a livelihood: "it had become a passion." Such a strong interpretation is supported by equally strong evidence. Gordon refused to close her clinic when threatened with legal sanctions for violating local laws that restricted the sale of birth control devices to doctors and pharmacists. Rather, she reworked her fee structure. Gordon sold only her advice; birth control devices were free of charge. Gradually, each paragraph—begun with an assertion (or interpretation) and built with data for a reader to consider—builds toward support of Holz's overarching story. The birth control movement in America, she argues, was not only built by nationally known nurses such as Margaret Sanger. It was also built by other less well-known but equally committed ones such as Gordon working in communities and clinics all across the United States.

It is stories such as those told by historians like Holz about nurses like Gordon that capture the essence of what history is and what its conceptual and methodological issues seek to address. History is, as Howell and Prevenier (2001) write, "the stories we tell about our prior selves or those that others tell about us" (p. 1). And its conceptual and methodological framework structures the choices we make as we create such stories. We have, to date, told many fascinating and important stories that have created collective meanings and memories for a quite disparate group of professionals. And we have many more such stories to tell. So—get reading, get researching, and, above all, "*get writing.*"

REFERENCES

Abel, E. (1994). Family caregiving in the 19th century: Emily Hawley Gillespie and Sarah Gillespie Huftalen, 1858–1888. *Bulletin of the History of Medicine, 68,* 573–599.

Boschma, G. (1999). High ideals versus harsh reality: A historical analysis of mental health nursing in Dutch asylums, 1890–1920. *Nursing History Review, 7,* 127–151.

Buck, J. (2007). Reweaving a tapestry of care: Religion, nursing, and the meaning of hospice, 1945–1978. *Nursing History Review, 15,* 113–145.

Carr, E. H. (1961). *What is history?* New York: Vintage Books.

Choy, C. (2003). *Empire of care: Nursing and migration in Filipino American history.* Durham and London: Duke University Press, 1–14.

Crowder, E. (2006). *Passing the legacy: The last fifty years of the School of Nursing at the hospital of the University of Pennsylvania.* Philadelphia: The Alumni Association of the Hospital of the University of Pennsylvania School of Nursing.

D'Antonio, P. (1999). Revisiting and rethinking the rewriting of nursing history. *Bulletin of the History of Medicine, 73,* 269.

D'Antonio, P. (2006). History for a practice profession. *Nursing Inquiry, 13*(4), 242–248.

Fairman, J. (1999). Delegated by default or negotiated by need: Physicians, nurse practitioners, and the process of clinical thinking. *Medical Humanities Review, 13*(1), 38–58.

Fischer, D. H. (1970). *Historians' fallacies: Toward a logic of historical thought.* New York: Harper Torchbooks.

Forman, P. (1991). Independence, not transcendence, for the historian of science. *ISIS, 82,* 71–86.

Gaddis, J. L. (2002). *The landscape of history: How historians map the past.* New York: Oxford University Press.

Holz, R. (2005). Nurse Gordon on trial: Those early days of the birth control movement reconsidered. *Journal of Social History, 39*(1), 112–140.

Howell, M., & Prevenier, W. (2001). *From reliable sources: An introduction to historical methods.* Ithaca, NY: Cornell University Press.

Keeling, A. (2004). Blurring the boundary between medicine and nursing: Coronary care nursing, circa the 1960s. *Nursing History Review, 12,* 139–165.

King, N. (2006). *Writing up your study.* Retrieved December 30, 2006, from http://www.hud.ac.uk/hhs/research/template_analysis/technique/writingup.htm

Kocka, J. (1996). What is leftist about social history today. *Journal of Social History, 29*(Special Suppl.), 67–71.

Kocka, J. (2003). Losses, gains and opportunities: Social history today. *Journal of Social History, 37*(1), 21–28.

Magnússon, S. G. (2003). The singularization of history: Social history and microhistory within the postmodern state of knowledge. *Journal of Social History, 36*(3), 701–735.

Rafferty, A. M., & Solano, D. (2007). The rise and demise of the colonial nursing service: British nurses in the colonies, 1896–1966. *Nursing History Review, 15,* 147–154.

Reverby, S. (1989). *Ordered to care: The dilemma of American nursing: 1860–1945.* New York: Cambridge University Press.

Sandelowski, M. (2000). The physician's eyes: American nursing and the diagnostic revolution in medicine. *Nursing History Review, 8,* 3–38.

Shkimba, M., & Flynn, K. (2005). In England we did nursing: Caribbean and British nurses in Great Britain and Canada, 1950–1970. In B. Mortimer & S. McGann (Eds.), *New directions in the history of nursing: International perspectives* (pp. 141–157). London: Routledge.

Storey Kelleher, W. (2004). *Writing history: A guide for students* (2nd ed., p. 61). New York: Oxford University Press.

Sweet, H. (2004). "Wanted: 16 nurses of the better educated type": Provision of nurses to South Africa in the late 19th and early 20th centuries. *Nursing Inquiry, 11*(3), 176–184.

Wikipedia. *Samuel Eliot Morison Biography.* Retrieved March 3, 2007, from http://en.wikipedia.org/wiki/Samuel_Eliot_Morison

CHAPTER THREE

Doing Historical Research

Sandra B. Lewenson

History provides ways of knowing and understanding events, people, places, and issues. Historians study history to explain what happened in the past. They seek clarity of the past that is replete with ambiguity, conflicting stories, and confusing relationships between and among variables (Lynaugh & Reverby, 1987). These variables may consist of social, political, economic, racial, gender, professional, and other factors that help to explain the topic under investigation. Examining history, specifically nursing history, leads to and supports better decision making in health care. Decision making in nursing requires a critical understanding of historical antecedents. This understanding provides decision makers with a greater depth and breadth of knowledge that will ultimately better inform their decisions (Lewenson, in press). D'Antonio (2004) writes that history may serve as a "new paradigm for nursing knowledge" (p. 1). This knowledge can best be gained through historical research that systematically and simultaneously questions, explores, analyzes, critiques, and narrates the story. Historiography enables nurses to rethink and thus engage in rewriting nursing history (Davies, 2007). Interpreting historical data from different perspectives offers a variety of ways in which to explain and understand the phenomena under study.

STEPS IN GETTING STARTED

In order to gain an understanding of nursing history, knowing historical methodology is essential. Other chapters in *Capturing Nursing*

History: A Guide to Historical Methods in Research present the rationale for studying nursing history, the various frameworks that can be used, and a host of other issues surrounding historiography. This chapter focuses specifically on the process of doing historical research. The overwhelming question of "how do I begin?" becomes more manageable when you understand and examine the steps of what goes into the process of historical research. To do this, this chapter uses case studies to explain the steps involved in historical research, explore the thinking involved in these steps, and, most importantly, raise the questions that guide the historical research.

While this chapter provides "steps" in doing historical research, these steps provide a guide, and only a guide. Steps can be completed in any order—systematically, simultaneously, and even chaotically. Many authors who write about doing historiography explain that there is no one method to use; however, similarities in the approach exist (Lusk, 1997; Lynaugh & Reverby, 1987). Lusk (1997) writes about the stages that most historians go through, such as "choosing a topic and an appropriate theoretical framework, finding and accessing the sources, analyzing, synthesizing, interpreting and reporting the data" (p. 355). Using similar stages, Lewenson (2007b) provides historical researchers with a guide to completing historical research that has been adapted for this chapter (see Table 3.1). As Lynaugh and Reverby (1987) explain, there is no one method to complete historical research, just guideposts that lead the researcher.

Table 3.1 outlines the steps involved in historical research as guideposts for historians to use. Each item is bulleted rather than numbered to remove the idea of a specific step-by-step order. This chapter explains what each step involves and highlights these steps with material from case studies. The case studies interspersed throughout the steps illustrate the experience of this author as well as that of other historians. These steps give form and meaning to the experiences of historians, thus providing examples of organizing schematics that attempt to assist those interested in capturing nursing history.

TABLE 3.1 Steps in "Doing" Historical Research

- Identify Area of Interest
- Raise Questions
- Formulate Title
- Review Literature
- Interpret Data
- Write the Narrative

Table adapted from Lewenson, 2007b, pp. 274–275.

Identify an Area of Interest

To begin a historical study, identify an area of interest. Think about why you are interested in the subject you selected. This interest usually develops organically from your experiences, such as a job, a class, a trip, or a book. Ask yourself, "What led me to examine this area?" "What do I hope to learn by investigating the history of this area of interest?" and "What are the 'bigger' questions surrounding the area of interest?" Reflecting on who you are also provides you, the researcher, with a better understanding of why you chose the topic you did. Acknowledging who you are may give you a better sense of direction as you proceed through the investigation. Who you are as a researcher has an impact on the work you do as a historian. Rafferty (1997/1998) explains that an author's politics and values shape the method and the "interpretive approach to data analysis" (p. 9). Thus, spending time to self-reflect may provide you with the insights that will alert you to the types of frameworks you will use, the way you may interpret the data, and the narrative you will write.

Consider a historical study as a work in progress. Historians raise questions and find answers, only to raise more questions. Pajunen (1985) wrote in an editorial that "the wisdom and judgment of one historian ideally can prompt further questions" (p. 6). One's own questions and that of others who read the research will continue to push the boundaries of historical knowledge and understanding. Looking at the data from various perspectives creates different meanings and ways of understanding that can change as the researchers change their view. Historical research requires the ability to live not only with the ambiguity that Lynaugh and Reverby (1987) identify, but also with fluidity of ideas and meanings. Fluidity of thought creates meaningful ideas, but it also can create discomfort, which can be productive if one can accept it.

In the following section, I examine my own background as a way of identifying my interest in a study that I am currently engaged in. The study, tentatively titled "The Phasing Out of the Bellevue and Mills Schools of Nursing and the Expansion of Hunter College Department of Nursing, 1967," grew out of my own interest in the nursing school I had attended between 1967 and 1971.

Case Study

For years I have been interested in nursing education and why there seems to be so much conflict surrounding the "level of entry into practice" question. I have spent over 20 years in higher education, including 3 years as Director of Accreditation at the National League for Nursing, over 8 years as an Associate Dean, and several more years as full-time faculty. My interest in baccalaureate and higher education for nurses stems from my past as well as the many professional influences along the way. I return to my past to explore why I select the topics that I study.

I grew up in the Bronx in a family that valued higher education. Both my parents attended college, so when I said I wanted to become a nurse, the only way my parents would support my goal was to have me enroll in a baccalaureate program. Little did we know that the decision to enter a 4-year program instead of a 2-year associate degree or a diploma program resonated with the 1965 ANA proposal for baccalaureate education.

I entered Hunter College–Bellevue School of Nursing in 1967, the first year that Bellevue School of Nursing (officially known as the Bellevue and Mills Schools of Nursing, Mills being the school of nursing for men) "phased-out" its widely acclaimed 3-year diploma program. Considered one of the first Nightingale-influenced training schools to open in the United States, the school established at Bellevue Hospital in New York City opened in 1873 (Dock & Stewart, 1938, p. 152). The history of the Bellevue School of Nursing reflected innovative thinking in nursing education. The Hunter students moved into the Bellevue nurses' residence at 440 East 26th Street and lived together (but on separate floors) with the last two classes of Bellevue's School of Nursing. While the Bellevue students enjoyed the reputation of being more clinically experienced, and perhaps more competent in their skills, Hunter students enjoyed the college experience. During my 4 years at Hunter–Bellevue, the women's movement, Vietnam War protests, and civil rights simultaneously added to my educational experiences at school. Many in my class marched in protest of social and political injustice, whereas the Bellevue nursing students were seemingly less visible, if present at all, at these extracurricular college activities. Our 2 days of clinical practice and many more hours in the classroom seemed to markedly contrast with the education of the Bellevue students. The "tension" between the two groups may have been more imagined than real, as I could hardly remember such tension other than hearing about it after graduation. Yet, the memories of Bellevue and Hunter alumnae may be different from my own and ones that cloud the vision of what may have really happened to make the dramatic change in educational levels and educational experiences for students. I can use the memories of my own experience at Hunter–Bellevue to raise questions and to explore the data.

Raise Questions

Throughout the process of historical research, one must ask questions. Questions raised by your own interest in the subject may begin the process. They help to focus your study, but need not limit your study. As one pursues the rationale and significance of the topic, additional questions emerge that direct the search for answers. The review of the literature, the search for evidence, and the way you organize the data influence and reflect the kind of questions that you raise. These questions will in turn guide the search for evidence, the interpretation of the data, and the narration of the story.

The kinds of funding sources that you may seek can also influence your questions and thus the thrust of the historical research. Is the funding source interested in ethical issues, underserved populations, or focused on how variables such as race, gender, or ethnicity affect the data? These questions often lead the researchers to refocus their study and look at other issues that might not have arisen without outside forces raising these questions.

Completing an Institutional Review Board (IRB) application required by most universities, colleges, and institutions forces the researchers to ask questions about the ethical issues in their study. How will you, the researcher, approach the data? Will you use archival collections or will you use private letters and papers that may raise ethical questions as to whether permission has been granted to use such materials? If you are interested in collecting oral histories, what kind of permissions do you need to obtain? Consider how you will use the data collected and where it will be stored in the future.

Keeping an open mind as you reflect on who you are, the readings you pursue, the grant applications, the Institutional Review Board applications, the rationale, and the purpose of the study will enable you to raise appropriate questions to direct your study. The questions you raise will also help to focus your study and isolate your subject from a larger whole, as Austin (1958) suggested. By isolating some part of the topic, your study usually becomes more manageable. Yet, you as a researcher need to be aware of this split so that you can then ultimately relate to the whole in the analysis and answer the important questions of "so what?" and "who cares?" These questions must be raised in order to make sense of why your work is relevant and meaningful to a larger audience.

The audience you write for influences the questions you may ask as well. Consider an audience who is interested in celebrating the first 100 years of their school's history. This group may be more interested in the celebratory nature of the history rather than a critique of the educational experiences in comparison with another school. The following case study reflects some of the questions I have raised in my current research of the Hunter–Bellevue School of Nursing.

Case Study

I often wondered why Bellevue Hospital's premiere school, a 3-year diploma program, phased out its program to allow a 4-year degree-granting program to expand in its place. Why give up something that was working? Or was it not working? Why did Hunter College expand its program at Bellevue, and what made them change from a department to a School of Nursing? Why was Hunter College chosen to expand its school at Bellevue instead of another school like New York University that already had a link with educating Bellevue students at the baccalaureate level? Who were the people involved that made these changes, and why? Some of these questions I could not formulate until I began to read through the minutes of the meetings of Hunter and Bellevue faculty and administrators.

I knew some of the Hunter students from my own experience, but I wondered how we looked demographically as a class? What made our class different from the diploma students who entered the 3-year degree program? Were diploma students from different socioeconomic, political, racial, ethnic, or religious backgrounds? Were they from the five New York City boroughs as most, if not all, of the Hunter students were? At Hunter there was no tuition, compliments of the City of New York. All one had to be was a New York City resident to qualify for the free tuition. Did Bellevue students come from across the country, from different backgrounds, or were the students mostly from the New York metropolitan region? And, if we were from different backgrounds, did this make a difference in the nurses we became?

In the beginning of my research, I applied for funding. While I was unsuccessful in obtaining the grant funding, the process of writing the application helped to formulate my ideas and raise further questions for the study. One of the most important questions that I raised, with the help of the person sponsoring the funding source, was "what was the larger issue?" My conversation with her forced me to consider what I really was studying and what I was really questioning. Was it about Hunter–Bellevue's merger? My own experience in nursing school? The issue of baccalaureate entry into practice? Or could it have something to do with who went to nursing school and how the change in educational levels changed the demographic makeup of the student body and, ultimately, the nurses who graduated? I continued to try to answer the important questions of so what, and who cares? Why should we care what happened when Bellevue's leadership phased out its school? How did Bellevue respond to the 1965 ANA proposal that called for a baccalaureate degree for entry into practice, but never fully influenced such an educational outcome? Was the change in Bellevue generated by academic reasons or purely financial? Was it too costly for Bellevue, a city hospital, to operate a nursing school during the fiscally difficult years of the 1960s? Who were the leaders at Hunter, and what did they want from Bellevue's past? What did Hunter seek by expanding into Bellevue's building? The questions kept emerging and began to focus my study.

Formulate Title

Formulate a title for your study, but be prepared to change it many times. The title simply tells the reader what the study is about. It provides an opening glimpse of what you studied, why you studied it, and the years you studied. The title both focuses you, the researcher, and informs the consumer of the research about the study. The title should entice the audience to read the study and can reflect the researcher's sense of creativity and humor. Often titles reflect key thoughts or quotes from the study itself, such as "The Ultimate Destination of All Nursing": The Development of District Nursing in England, 1880–1925 (Howse, 2007) and "Much Instruction Needed Here": The Work of Nurses in Rural Wisconsin During the Depression (Apple, 2007). One of the pitfalls of an overly creative title occurs when the reader tries to find a historical study by searching an electronic database or Internet source and cannot find the study because the first few words of the title do not reflect the topic. If the first few words do not direct the search to the topic, the study may lose its potential impact on a large number of readers.

Case Study

In the first 3 months of my study about Hunter–Bellevue School of Nursing, I changed the title several times. First, I called the study the Closing of Bellevue Training School for Nurses and Opening of Hunter–Bellevue School of Nursing, 1967. That was before I began the review of primary sources and meeting with Mary Tomaselli, the Administrator of the Alumnae Association of the Bellevue School of Nursing. It was explained to me that Bellevue was never *closed,* but instead the term *phased out* was used. This distinction in terms was important and may have related to the accreditation of Bellevue's School of Nursing. Hunter College did not take over and become the new Bellevue School of Nursing. Instead, Hunter had expanded its own program that had begun in 1943. By expanding into the Bellevue facility, the department of Nursing Education at Hunter College, under the leadership of Marguerite C. Holmes, increased the number of students in 1967 and became a School of Nursing at Hunter College, part of the City University of New York (CUNY) system. With Mary Tomaselli's help, I corrected the language in my initial title to more accurately reflect what had happened.

I then tried catchier, more interesting versions of a title, for example, " 'When One Door Closes, Another Opens': The History of the 'Phasing Out' of Bellevue School of Nursing and the Opening of Hunter–Bellevue School of Nursing." But, if one were to do an electronic database search, they would find nothing with this title (as in the case of CINAHL). Or, in a search on Google, you would be directed to the direct quote attributed to Alexander Graham Bell, Helen Keller, and other famous writers.

I continued to work at the title to include the elements of the major focus of the study, and to be as accurate as possible. While I still only have a working title, and it will most likely change several times over, the latest rendition is, "The History of the 'Phasing Out' of Bellevue and Mills Schools of Nursing and the Expansion of the Hunter College Department of Nursing Education at Bellevue, 1967." (I included Mills School in the title as that was Bellevue's school for men, and I want to be sure to look at Mill's role in the *phasing out.* Also, from the materials I have read to date, the complete title for the school at Bellevue was the Bellevue and Mills Schools of Nursing. Additionally, if I am looking at gender, it would be important to include the Mills School of Nursing in this study.)

Review Literature

A review of the literature is an ongoing event that starts with the identified interest in the topic, responds to the questions that you raise, and focuses on the factors and years you identify in the working title. The literature review also prompts more questions that the researcher may want to respond to and influences the title itself. This step continues throughout the research and continually feeds the ongoing process. Starting the literature review begins with immersing yourself in the area of interest through finding the primary and secondary sources that will direct you in the study. This chapter focuses on the types of source material available. It does not go into depth about where one finds these sources, but discussion about archives can be found in other chapters within *Capturing Nursing History.*

Secondary Sources

Secondary sources provide depth and meaning to a topic. They inform the researchers' understanding of what has been written before about the subject. One source can provide the names of other sources that can and perhaps should be reviewed. Reading, as noted by D'Antonio (2005), is an essential element of historical research, and this is especially true during the literature review. Reading various works about a subject affords the researcher a broader understanding of the contextual factors involved in the study.

The literature review takes on a life of its own as the researcher tries to fully understand the subject. Lusk (1997) explains how the "background reading also brings richness and depth to a subject, faintly coloring in the fabric of the diverse ephemera of daily life and adding complexity and realism." More pragmatically, Lusk explains that a "thorough knowledge of the context and details of a subject can save researchers and archivists time, frustration, and expense (p. 1 of Gale Group, or p. 355 in the original article). During the literature review, secondary sources help to refine the questions, direct the study, and enhance the understanding of the subject under investigation.

Case Study

The literature review for my current research started with my first historical study, and perhaps even before that. When I worked on an earlier study titled "'Taking Charge': Nursing, Suffrage, and Feminism, 1873–1920," I explored the many well-documented historiographies about the history of nursing in the United States. These historiographies were written by noted historians in the 1970s and 1980s, such as "'The Physician's Hand': Work, Culture, and Conflict in American Nursing" by Barbara Melosh (1982); "'Ordered to Care': The Dilemma of American Nursing 1850–1945" by Susan Reverby (1987); and "Hospitals, Paternalism, and the Role of the Nurse" by JoAnn Ashley (1976). I also examined the work of earlier nurse historians such as Lavinia Dock and Isabel Stewart's (1938) work on the history of nursing. I read articles published in nursing journals throughout the 20th century to help me understand nursing education, political activity, and the changing image of nurses. I was struck by the number of secondary sources that provided various ways of thinking and knowing about nursing's professional development during the late 19th and early 20th centuries. The readings answered some questions, but typically raised more. The readings helped me organize my ideas about my study. I was interested in the feminist perspective and viewed the nursing profession's development through this lens. In addition, the sociopolitical experiences of the period in which nursing moved toward professionalization added another dimension to the way I approached the data and thus interpreted the findings.

During my current study, I am building on my past reviews of literature and knowledge of the period, as well as adding other readings pertaining to the development of nursing education in the United States. For my current literature review, I am reading works such as *A Curriculum Guide for Schools of Nursing* (published by the Committee on Curriculum of the National League of Nursing Education in 1937) and *Nursing for the Future* (Brown, 1948).

I am in the process of collecting and reading articles written during the 1940s, 1950s, and 1960s about nursing education and the response nursing had toward the American Nurses Association position on baccalaureate education in nursing. I found the database JSTOR extremely helpful in identifying journal articles from the *American Journal of Nursing* spanning back to 1900 when the journal first was published. The use of technology has been especially helpful during this study. For example, library database searches and Google searches for archival material speed up the process of identifying where, who, what, and how to find both primary and secondary sources. The American Association for the History of Nursing Web site (http://www.aahn.org) also serves as an excellent resource for accessing information about various sources.

In this study, I am also interested in the sociopolitical activities of nurses and the connection with the ideas of feminism of the 1960s. The reading for this study builds on some of my earlier work looking at nursing political relationship with the women's movement, nursism, and accreditation. I continue to seek out the writing that was produced during the mid-20th century to help me contextualize my current research and identify additional primary source possibilities.

Primary Sources

Historical studies need primary sources. These sources provide firsthand accounts that can offer the historian important insight into a particular period, event, or person's life. Primary sources supply evidence to past experiences. Yet, the primary sources, such as letters, diaries, and minutes of meetings, lack critical analysis and often contain the bias of the original author of those sources. The historical researcher must critically analyze the primary sources used in their study (Lewenson, 2007a, 2007b). This analysis is framed by the theoretical framework, the knowledge gleaned from other primary and secondary sources, the researcher's knowledge of the context in which the primary sources were written, the researcher's own bias, and a variety of methodological issues and limitations of historical research. Among these limitations are missing, confusing, and ambiguous data, a lack of perspective, and questions about the genuineness and authenticity (Lewenson, 2007a, 2007b).

Historians must consider the genuineness and authenticity of the primary sources. Are they really what they purport to be, and do they make sense given the time period in which the materials were found? Barzun and Graff (1985) explain that for a document to be genuine, the document is what it says it is. If the primary sources contain minutes written by Lavinia Dock, then Dock would need to have been the author of these records. Authenticity refers to the idea that the document provides a truthful reporting of the subject (Barzun & Graff, 1985). It is the historian's responsibility to assure that primary source data are what they say they are and provide a truthful account. For example, once, while reading the minutes of the American Society of Superintendents of Training School (called the National League for Nursing), I remember a brief discussion about the purchase of a typewriter. After having read through the long hand-written minutes of the organization since it first began in 1893, I was delighted to note on one of my index cards the following: "at last minutes were finally typed starting November 13, 1909." The request for a typewriter apparently had been approved, and a typewriter had been purchased. This request was appropriate for the period of time, but had the secretary asked for a computer, the truthfulness of the data would have been questioned.

Authenticating sources can be daunting when using material found outside of archival collections, such as letters found in a storeroom of a hospital or your aunt's attic. Barzun and Graff (1985) explain that to assure the validity of their resources, researchers may rely on "attention to detail, on common-sense reasoning, on a 'developed' field for history and chronology, on familiarity with human behavior, and on ever-enlarging stores of information" (p. 112).

Primary sources crucial to historical research provide evidence that must be explored using various perspectives. Mansell (1999) writes about the concern that primary sources may provide only one side of an issue and therefore may be considered part of a methodological limitation. Mansell uses the organizational records in Canada as an example. These records, Mansell said, do not portray the life of the "rank and file" in nursing and thus serve to limit the response to the research questions about "class, status, and ethnicity" of these nurses as opposed to the leadership in nursing (p. 220). Using a combination of primary sources including oral histories, however, provide a more "complete story" to unfold (p. 221).

Use of oral histories as primary sources also adds to the tools of the historian. Norman (2002) writes about her early experience doing historical research. Not finding primary source material about the veteran Vietnam War nurses, she "decided to record and analyze these nurses' experiences" (p. 122). Oral histories, discussed in more detail in later chapters in this book, provide important firsthand accounts of events, life experiences, and data that need to be collected. Here, too, oral history must be analyzed within the context of the whole, knowing that bias exists within the data that must be accounted for in the interpretation.

When discussing primary sources, researchers must also think about what types of primary sources they will use, as well as the location of those records. Archives contain many of the primary sources that researchers use, such as letters, memoirs, diaries, organizational minutes, speeches, and other important papers. Considering where primary sources are located and accessing these collections is central to the research process. There may be a cost involved in travel to the archives, and the distinct nature of the archives, as opposed to a library search, requires the researcher to take time to assess how to approach their use.

Archives were the topic of discussion at the American Association for the History of Nursing archives preconference in 2004. There, Rafferty (2004) spoke of the intimate relationship that can develop between the historian and the primary source material when handling the documents. The feel of the paper, the content of the material, and the quiet sound of the archives may all contribute to this developing relationship. Reading the letters of Lavinia Dock or Lillian Wald, for example, can foster a more personal relationship with the author of the letters. I cried when I read a newspaper clipping found in the archives that Isabel Hampton Robb had died an untimely death. Even though I knew the circumstances surrounding her death, reading a news account in the archives made it all too real. Lorentzon (2004) also compares the reassurance that touching and smelling musty paper archives has in comparison with the "coldness" experienced by researchers using microfilm readers and computer screens (p. 280).

Case Study

The primary source material I am using can be found in a variety of archives and on site at the Hunter–Bellevue School of Nursing. I identified some of these sources following conversations with the Director of the School of Nursing, Diane Rendón, who is both an alumna of the Bellevue School of Nursing as well as the Director of Hunter's nursing program. She connected me with Mary Tomaselli, the Administrator of the Alumnae Association of the Bellevue School of Nursing, and to the records still retained on the premises of the school about the expansion of Hunter College in 1967. Mary Tomaselli granted me access to pertinent records still remaining in the alumnae office, such as the folder containing minutes from the Executive Committee of the Bellevue Schools of Nursing, 1953–1969. Most of the Bellevue and Mills Schools of Nursing material is already housed at the Foundation of New York State Nurses where I will eventually go to review them. However, I do love using the documents directly from the files at the school. These are historic documents that have not yet made it to the archives.

As I continue my study, I plan to examine the archival records of the American Nurses Association located at the Mugar Library and the National League for Nursing located at the National Library of Medicine. My purpose in seeking out these primary sources is to examine the broader issues of why the many educational levels of entry into nursing practice continue, what this means in terms of how nursing is valued in society, and the effect on the nursing profession's ability to serve the public.

I also plan to collect oral histories of former faculty and students of the Bellevue and Mills Schools and Hunter College–Bellevue School of Nursing to understand what their thoughts were related to the phasing out of Bellevue and Mills School of Nursing and the expansion of Hunter College. These oral histories will serve as part of the primary source material for this study. I have already completed an IRB review that addresses the ethical concerns surrounding the use of oral histories. In addition, as part of the IRB process, a decision about the disposition of the oral histories following the studies completion was made. These oral histories will become part of an archival collection, most likely housed at the Foundation of the New State York Nurses in Guilderland, New York.

I have begun collecting oral histories using an IPod digital recorder rather than a tape recorder. The benefits of digital recording far outweigh (for me) the use of a tape recorder. The voices sound clearer, I can save the recordings directly on the computer, the size of the IPod is smaller than the tape recorder, and I never have to stop the interview to turn the tape. My biggest concern is still finding an appropriate person to do the transcriptions as well as finding funding to support the cost of doing the oral histories. Some of the costs I need to consider include the cost of the equipment, travel, and transcription.

My search for primary sources may lead me to examine documents of other diploma schools of nursing that closed in the 1960s or soon after. I am searching for sources that will help to uncover any shared similarities with the academic shift at Bellevue. I also plan to examine the papers of nursing leaders such as Eleanor Lambertsen, Francis Reiter, Theresa Lynch, and others that may shed light on the tenor of the period in which I am studying. I keep my mind open to additional possibilities where primary sources may be found and welcome further dialogue, readings, and opportunities to talk with others about this process.

Interpret Data

Lynaugh (1998) wrote that "history is like real life; it is contingent. Science necessarily tries to control contingencies; historians must include them in their analysis" (p. 1). Interpreting data entails using creativity to examine the data, placing the data within a context, and making the connections between and among the variables in data. Contingencies, like Lynaugh suggests, are taken into account as the researcher interprets the data.

Some of the contingencies that historians deal with include conflicting stories, missing pieces, personal and professional bias and ideology, and various organizing frameworks, to name but a few. Rafferty (1997/1998) stated that historians "work within the compass of evidential resources and primary sources of data preserved by posterity" (p. 6). The sources may be incomplete, ambiguous, and conflicting, yet, historians work around these issues and make decisions about the data. Organizing the evidence preserved by posterity is necessary in order to place the data, whatever data there is, in some form of contextual framework. The contextual framework may be the use of a feminist perspective, a sociopolitical framework, or a biographical framework that enables the researcher to "put their arms around the material," in some form of logical, coherent way. In biographies, for example, one can see the connections made between the individual being studied and the larger context in which the individual lives. Biography affords historians opportunity to better understand the "connections made between and among the individuals who shape the history of nursing" (Lewenson, 2006, p. 2). The historian uses the primary sources as evidence and works with the various contingencies to make sense of the data.

The researcher's ideas and ideologies influence the framework used and the interpretation of the evidence (Rafferty, 1997/1998). The researcher's bias comes into play here influencing the way the data are examined, organized, and explained. Self-reflection assists the researcher address this concern and allows for a more truthful interpretation of the data (Austin, 1958; Barzun & Graff, 1985; Lewenson, 2007a).

Christy (1978) wrote that, "healthy skepticism becomes a way of life for the serious historiographer" (p. 7). Researchers deal with a variety of conflicting truths in order to find meaning in the data. Balance between the differences in the data becomes an important task of the historian (Lewenson, 2007a; Tholfsen, 1977). In this step, as in previous ones, questions need to be addressed about the content found in the primary and secondary sources, such as the congruency of the data and the possible conflicting stories. The historian looks for the conflict as part of the healthy skepticism and tries to justify the findings.

Case Study

How I will interpret the data in my current study, "Phasing Out," is still yet to be determined. I am in the early stage of the research process and am identifying the kind of sources I need to find and where they may be found. I have yet to frame the research data, but my hunch is that I will be looking at the data from a sociopolitical framework. The influence of growing up in the 1950s and 1960s, my interest in higher education and women's rights, and the work of my previous study will be reflected in the framework I select and in the subsequent interpretation of the data. My personal and professional biases will be reflected and will have to be acknowledged as well. I am also interested in the contextual factors that may have influenced the phasing out of Bellevue and Hunter's expansion.

I have started to collect data and have heard an interesting story that illustrates the notion of conflicting stories and the need to understand what the "truth" might be. In a personal conversation on January 30, 2007, Mary Tomaselli and I spoke about how the Bellevue alumni had been surveyed as to whether or not they would permit Hunter students to wear the Bellevue nursing cap. Mary gave me a copy of an article published in the *Bellevue Bulletin* about her understanding of the issue. Over 3,427 Bellevue alumnae had opposed the use of the Bellevue cap by Hunter students with only 288 voting in favor and 3 who voted neutral (Tomaselli, 1970). The memory that Bellevue would not permit Hunter students to wear the famed Bellevue cap seemed to serve as a source of conflict for some of the Hunter students and a sense of pride for the Bellevue students. Yet, as Tomaselli noted, the Chairman of Hunter's program, Marguerite C. Holmes, did not want Hunter students to wear Bellevue's cap because Hunter already had their own cap, a cap that the school had used for over 20 years. Nor, apparently, was there evidence that the Hunter students or alumnae had requested the Bellevue cap. This was a concern more of the Bellevue Board of Managers than of the students or faculty of Bellevue or Hunter. Seemingly, the "myth" about Hunter students wanting to wear the Bellevue cap took on a life of its own. The veracity needed to be determined as to the truthfulness of the incidence, why it may have happened, and what the ramifications, if any, were on the phasing out of Bellevue's School of Nursing and the expansion of the Hunter College Department of Nursing.

Write the Narrative

This step in the historical research process requires the historian to tell the story. The story unfolds, highlighting the findings, answering the questions, showing the conflicts, explaining the ambiguities, and bracketing the biases. The historical narrative should capture the audiences' interest and hold their attention. This requires the historical researcher to switch from a passive voice and make connections with the data that relay clear, interesting human connections (Lynaugh, 2000). Lynaugh's editorial in *Nursing History Review* captures the essence of what the narrative requires. Lynaugh wrote:

> the history of nursing is full of unique and fascinating events and people; our subject is not dull. I think the task of writing is to make the narrative live for the reader in the same way it thrills us as we discover it. Good history tells the whole story, usually in a chronological fashion

> with a beginning, middle, and end. It is a big challenge to set the time, get the facts right and in their proper context, and to do it in such a way that the reader clings to the story. (p. 1)

The narrative presents the whole study to the reader. In the telling of the story, the historian responds to the questions raised during the research process, identifies the primary and secondary sources, connects the ideas together, and shares any of the concerns raised by the interpretation of the data. All this while engaging the reader in a suspenseful, dramatic, and meaningful account of the topic under study. This part of the historical research process may be the most difficult to successfully complete. Comfort with words to creatively weave the events, the ideas, the assumptions, the biases, the "aha's" gained from interpreting the evidence illustrates some of the difficulty that faces the historiographer at this stage of the process. Judgment of the study lies within the story line and how successful it was in pulling all the elements of the historiography together. For example, acceptance for publication and approval of the final product, in part, relates to the way the narrative can combine the various elements of the study and present a cogent story.

Shirley Fondiller (1978) writes that the way in which a researcher organizes the data will support the task of writing the narrative. She warns against collecting too much data, noting that "every researcher's fear of overlooking some splendid gem of historical import" (p. 26) can be an issue. Fondiller says to "Work with what you have" (p. 26) and organize using any number of ways to explain the story. For example, you can use a biographical, or chronological, or issue-based approach when writing the narrative.

Use of direct quotes from the primary sources adds humanness to the telling of the story. To hear Lavinia Dock or Lillian Wald speak out about social concerns of their day gives the reader a "close-up and personal" view of the time period when they expressed those words. Using direct quotes also can be an excellent way for the historian to provide "corroboration of and credibility" to their interpretation of the data (Lewenson, 2007a, p. 269).

In this next case study, I share my own thoughts about my research into the phasing out and the expansion of the two schools of nursing being studied and how I will shape the narrative to be interesting, informative, creative, and scholarly.

Case Study

Capturing the interest of the readers will be a challenge. Why is the story about one school's closing and the expansion of another interesting to the reader? Regardless of the audience, how will the drama unfold, the myths unravel, and the relevance of the study reveal itself? I will look for interesting quotes and anecdotes that may put a human face on the story. Using a chronological ordering of the data to tell the story about nursing education, social and political events of the mid-20th century, and nursing's response to these changes will all become mixed with the stories from the people who lived before, through, and after the phasing out and expansion of the schools. I will look to the letters and records of both schools as well as the oral histories for direct quotes that will tell the story from the perspective of those who lived through the experiences.

Where do I start the story for this study? Perhaps I will begin the narrative explaining the concern for a sufficient number of educated 21st-century nurses that will be able to meet the demands of the increasingly complex health care system. The story would unfold with the background history of nursing education in the United States, highlighting the mid-twentieth century studies. A chronological order would help organize the study, and chapters would be written around important events, for example: the history of nursing education in the United States (including several of the mid-twentieth century reports), the history of Bellevue and Mills Schools of Nursing, the history of nursing at Hunter College, the profession's move toward baccalaureate entry into practice, Bellevue's foresight and Hunter's expansion, what has happened since, and closing. My ideas about the telling of the story will change as I progress in the data collection. The analysis and synthesis of the data will inform the narrative I write, but for now, thinking about the possible organization helps guide me through the research process.

A word of caution needs to be made here. I must be careful to know when enough data are collected for this particular study. For my dissertation, I collected, and collected, and collected some more. When historian Nettie Birnbach found me at the *American Journal of Nursing* library surrounded by stacks of materials, she asked me about my study. Following my lengthy response, she urged me to stop and go home saying, "You are writing your dissertation, not your life's work!" She helped me understand that while I may not have covered all of the possibilities, it was time to go home, organize the data, and write.

CLOSING

Steps presented in this chapter barely scratch the surface of how to do historical research. Rafferty (1997/1998) argued "that historical research itself provides a useful method with which to unravel the experience of becoming both a researcher and an historian" (p. 6). By doing historical research, one learns the craft of historical research. In the process of doing, one needs to talk with others who are similarly engaged. Bounce ideas off each other, share your concerns about the method, and learn from each other. Find a mentor to work with who will read your material and listen to you while doing the research. Join groups, such as the American Association for the History of Nursing (AAHN), that provide an outlet for those learning about and doing historical research. Visit the AAHN Web site (http://www.aahn.org) for information about resources that can be used in the research process, such as a bibliography of historical methods, the listing of archival collections, and the listing of other historical associations that support the researcher. Attend history conferences and bring others with you. Access the various centers that support historical research in nursing. Enjoy the companionship of other historians, but also be ready to work alone, for it is with the primary and secondary sources, the archives, the data, and the computer that you will be sharing much of your time. Prepare to spend time reading about the historical method, for as stated in the beginning of this chapter there is no one way to do historical research, just guideposts along the way. And, most important, enjoy the process of doing historical research. The joy of discovery motivates many of us to continue to pursue this avenue of research.

REFERENCES

Apple, R. D. (2007). "Much instruction needed here": The work of nurses in rural Wisconsin during the depression. *Nursing History Review, 15*, 95–111.

Ashley, J. A. (1976). *Hospitals, paternalism, and the role of the nurse*. New York: Teachers College Press.

Austin, A. (1958). The historical method. *Nursing Research, 7*(1), 4–10.

Barzun, J., & Graff, H. F. (1985). *The modern researcher* (4th ed.). San Diego, CA: Harcourt Brace Jovanovich.

Brown, E. L. (1948). *Nursing for the future: A report for the National Nursing Council.* New York: Russell Sage Foundation.

Christy, T. (1978). The hope of history. In M. L. Fitzpatrick (Ed.), *Historical studies in nursing* (pp. 3–11). New York: Teachers College Press.

Committee on Curriculum of the National League of Nursing Education. (1937). *A curriculum guide for schools of nursing.* New York: National League of Nursing Education.

D'Antonio, P. (2004). Editor's note. *Nursing History Review, 12,* 1–3.

D'Antonio, P. (2005). Editor's note. *Nursing History Review, 13,* 1–3.

Davies, C. (2007). Rewriting nursing history—again? *Nursing History Review, 15*, 11–28.

Dock, L. L., & Stewart, I. M. (1938). *A short history of nursing: From the earliest times to the present day.* New York: G. P. Putnam's Sons.

Fondiller, S. (1978). Writing the report. In M. L. Fitzpatrick (Ed.), *Historical studies in nursing* (pp. 25–27). New York: Teachers College Press.

Howse, C. (2007). "The ultimate destination of all nursing": The development of district nursing in England, 1880–1925. *Nursing History Review, 15*, 65–94.

Lewenson, S. B. (2006). Connecting the dots: Biography shapes nursing history. *Nursing History Review, 14*, 2–4.

Lewenson, S. B. (2007a). Chapter 11: Historical research method. In H. J. Speziale & D. R. Carpenter (Eds.), *Qualitative research in nursing: Advancing the humanistic imperative* (4th ed., pp. 251–272). Philadelphia: Lippincott.

Lewenson, S. B. (2007b). Chapter 12: Historical research in practice, education, and administration. In H. J. Speziale & D. R. Carpenter (Eds.), *Qualitative research in nursing: Advancing the humanistic imperative* (4th ed., pp. 273–300). Philadelphia: Lippincott.

Lewenson, S. B. (2008). Looking back: History and decision-making. In S. B. Lewenson & M. Truglio-Londrigan (Eds.), *Decision-making in nursing: Thoughtful approaches for practice.* Boston: Jones & Bartlett, 13–28.

Lorentzon, M. (2004). Nursing Record/British Journal of Nursing archives, 1888–1956. *British Journal of Nursing, 13*(5), 280–284.

Lusk, B. (1997). Historical methodology for nursing research. *Image: Journal of Nursing Scholarship, 29*(4), 355–359 (reprint obtained through Gale Group, pp. 1–7).

Lynaugh, J. E. (1998). Editorial. *Nursing History Review, 6*, 1.

Lynaugh, J. E. (2000). Editorial. *Nursing History Review, 8*, 1.

Lynaugh, J., & Reverby, S. (1987). Thoughts on the nature of history. *Nursing Research, 36*(1), 4, 69.

Mansell, D. (1999). Sources in nursing historical research: A thorny methodological problem. *Canadian Journal of Nursing Research, 30*(4), 219–222.

Melosh, B. (1982). *"The physician's hand": Work, culture, and conflict in American nursing*. Philadelphia: Temple University Press.

Norman, B. (2002). Research vignette: The challenge of historical research. In G. LoBiondo-Wood & J. Haber (Eds.), *Nursing research: Methods, critical appraisal, and utilization* (5th ed., pp. 122–123). St. Louis: Mosby.

Pajunen, E. (1985). Editorial. *Journal of Nursing History, 1*(1), 5–6.

Rafferty, A. M. (1997/1998). Researching nursing's history: Writing, researching and reflexivity in nursing history. *Nurse Researcher, 5*(2), 5–16.

Rafferty, A. M. (2004). *Pre Conference.* Paper presented at the meeting of the American Association for the History of Nursing, Charleston, NC.

Reverby, S. (1987). *Ordered to care: The dilemma of American nursing 1850–1945.* Cambridge, UK: Cambridge University Press.

Tholfsen, T. R. (1977). The ambiguous virtues of the study of history. *Teachers College Record, 79*(2), 245–257.

Tomaselli, M. (1970, March). The Bellevue Cap. *Bellevue Bulletin* (Winter Issue), 13–14.

CHAPTER FOUR

Using Frameworks in Historical Research

Joy Buck

> Everything must be recaptured and relocated in the general framework of history, so that despite the difficulties, the fundamental paradoxes and contradictions, we may respect the unity of history which is also the unity of life.
>
> —Fernand Braudel, no date

Historians use a variety of tools and frameworks to help recapture and make sense out of the past. As historian Patricia D'Antonio points out in chapter 2, frameworks, such as social and political history, assist the historian in determining which questions will be asked, which data will be used for analysis, the processes by which such analyses will be conducted, and how these analyses will be contextualized in space and time. The practice of history has gone through changes over time, and the influence of the methods and theories of social, political, and cultural inquiry to its evolution during the 20th century has been significant (Howell & Prevenier, 2001; Novick, 1988).

Acknowledgments: This work was supported by the National Institute for Nursing Research: Individual National Research Service Award (F31 NR08301–01) and University of Virginia (2003–2005) and Advanced Training in Nursing Outcomes Research (T32-NR-007104) at the Center for Health Outcomes & Policy Research (2005–2007). I wish to thank my colleagues at the Center for Nursing Historical Inquiry and the Barbara Bates Center for the Study of the History of Nursing for their assistance in the development of this chapter and the essay "Hospice and the Politics of Terminal Care Reform in the United States" contained within.

SOCIAL FRAMEWORK

Until the 20th century, political history with its focus on "great white men" and "great events" dominated historical inquiry (Connolly, 2004; Lukacs, 2002; Novick, 1988). In the 20th century, however, the "great" historians of the past gave way to a new breed of historians with interests in studying the past from the "grass roots" or "bottom-up" rather than the "top-down." Social history provided an inclusive framework for reinterpreting the past and experiences of ordinary people, movements, and events through the thematic prisms of class, gender, and race (Lloyd, 1991; Stearns, 1983).

The "cross-disciplinary reciprocity" between history and the social sciences also influenced how historians studied and interpreted the work, worth, and education of nurses (D'Antonio, 1999). Consider for example, nurse historian Joan Lynaugh's (2006) use of a social framework in her analysis of which individuals and factors influenced the direction of nursing education during the latter half of the 20th century. Rather than privileging the acknowledged nursing leaders or "great women" of the day, Lynaugh focuses on the contributions of Mildred Tuttle, director of the Nursing Division of the W. K. Kellogg Foundation during the mid-20th century. Lynaugh suggests that Tuttle was a lesser known figure but nevertheless was an important player in the migration of nursing education from hospital training school into the university. As she points out, Tuttle was one of a small cadre of nurses who "seized the opportunity" to be central actors in shaping policy and allocating resources that resulted in "sweeping changes in how nurses were educated and in the very nature of nurses' work" (p. 204). While recognizing the continuity of enduring issues in nursing education over time, Lynaugh demonstrates that the possibility of change is very real.

CULTURAL FRAMEWORK

Another framework that emerged during the 20th century was that of cultural history. Cultural historians blend the approaches of history and anthropology to explore cultural interpretations of the past and cultural traditions in the present (Burke, 2004). Similar to social history, much of cultural history focuses on the shared experiences of the nonelite as expressed through public rituals and festivals, such as Mardi Gras in New Orleans, and the historical concepts of power, ideology, perception, cultural identity, and new historical narratives of body (Barzilai, 2003). The emphasis is not on just the behavior of groups or individuals, but rather the meaning behind these practices and their expression within the context and discourse of a given society at a particular point in time (Almond & Verba, 1965; Barzilai, 2003; Geertz, 1973; Kertzer, 1996).

An example of a study that examined the culture of nursing care within the broader historiographical framework of the Holocaust can be found in Barbara Brush's (2002) *Caring for Life: Nursing During the Holocaust.* Brush used oral and written testimonies of Jewish nurses during the Holocaust and their understanding and interpretation of nursing care in an environment that was antithetical to their training. Although not explicitly stated, Brush analyzed the interplay between a national policy and an extreme transition in nursing practice. For some of the nurses studied, the practice of nursing in the Jewish ghettoes and concentration camps was linked to self-preservation. The act of care provision served as a distancing tool to separate these nurses from the horrors surrounding them. As such, it offered a vehicle by which they could "preserve their own humanity through the moral treatment of others" (p. 78).

POLICY FRAMEWORK

While much of the 20th-century revisionist history steered clear of the political history of the past, by the mid-1970s, a group of historians argued that the study of social movements and the study of politics should not be mutually exclusive (Grossberg, 1979; Stearns & Tarr, 1993; Zelizer, 2005). The founding generation of policy historians included historians from within the academy who sought to use the past to inform present and future policy development and public historians outside who desired to generate history that was more accessible to a broader audience (Critchlow, 1993, 1998; Zelizer, 2000). In *Thinking in Time: The Uses of History for Decision Makers* (Neustadt & May, 1986), the authors demonstrate the various ways that history can, and in their view, should be utilized by policy makers and others involved in the policy process, from beginning to end. Despite an invigorated initial policy history movement, the use of policy as a framework to understand larger historical phenomena remained marginalized as a subfield in history. As one historian bemoaned in 1998, policy history was being taken over by the political and social scientists with a decidedly presentist tone (Critchlow, 1998, p. 459). A few years later, however, historian Julian Zelizer (2005) proclaimed that "the state of policy history is good" (p. 1).

A recent volume of essays edited by Rosemary Stevens, Charles Rosenberg, and Lawton Burns (2006) and a growing number of important studies attests the growth and vitality of this new subfield in history. When taken together, the essays in this volume expose how and why tensions between the competing forces of public need, professional agendas, and political expediency shaped interactions among health care institutions, health professionals, and recipients of care. The essays certainly build a strong argument for the role of history in answering some of the most vexing policy questions of contemporary times (Oliver, 2004; Oliver, Lee, & Lipton, 2004). Yet, the absence of a substantive analysis of the role of nursing—the largest of the health professions—in these essays and the vast majority of policy history literature is striking (Buck, 2007).

While scholarship on the politics of health policy is extensive (Fox, 1993; Gordon, 2004; Gottschalk, 2000; Marmor, 2000; Oberlander, 2003), very few studies have analyzed the tensions between and among top-down and bottom-up approaches to health care reform and the role of nurses and nursing within the policy arena (Diers, 2004; Mechanic & Reinhard, 2002). It is fortunate that a small number of nurse historians are examining the influence of nursing in the development of public policies and the impact of these policies on nursing (Brush, 2002; Brush & Berger, 2002; Brush, Sochalski, & Berger, 2004; Buck, 2004; Sampson, 2006). For example, Harriet Feldman and Sandra Lewenson (2000) used historical data to argue that nurses have in the past and continue to need to be front and center in policy development. Karen Buhler-Wilkerson's (2001) acclaimed history of home care proffers considerable insight into the persistence and political marginalization of nursing care for the sick at home during the 20th century. In doing so, she raises critical policy questions of who gets paid what for what type of care and where that care should be provided that are as relevant today as they were throughout much of the 20th century.

CASE STUDY USING A SOCIAL AND POLICY FRAMEWORK

My own work on the American hospice movement uses a combination of social and policy history frameworks to examine how and why the movement came about when it did and the ways in which the hospice philosophy of care was shaped as it was institutionalized (Buck, 2005). My interest in the history of hospice actually comes from my experiences as a clinician. I came to question why it was that there seemed to be such dissonances between the problems that I observed in the community, the types of care the patients and their families desired, and the policy solutions offered by politicians. Certainly, policy is heavily influenced by powerful interest groups, but the policy literature suggests that there are other factors as well. Political scientists characterize the American public and politicians as having no consistent, identifiable political ideology concerning health care or a health-related value system much beyond the idea of maintaining the status quo (Starr, 1982; Wing, 2000). They are risk averse and inclined toward symbolism, drama, and value-laden rhetoric (Buck, 2007; Weissert & Weissert, 2002). The policy cycle is short and the synergy of time, place, person, and circumstance are critical to the success of any policy option. As a historian, I am particularly interested in the dynamic interrelationships among and between these variables in time and across time. Thus, policy history offers an important methodological tool to help illuminate how and, more importantly, *why* certain policies were or were not adopted, as well as the impact of such actions or inactions. Drawing from my research on the development of hospice in the United States, some of which was published in *Nursing History Review* (Buck, 2004), the following essay offers another example of the saliency of policy history to our understanding of contemporary times.

Hospice and the Politics of Terminal Care Reform in the United States

When the renowned humorist Art Buchwald was diagnosed with end-stage renal disease in February 2006, he opted to forego renal dialysis and enter a hospice facility to spend what he and his physicians thought were the last days of his life. They were wrong. Buchwald spent the next 5 months in the hospice, eating whatever he pleased and holding court in the hospice's living room for his countless friends and dignitaries from around the world. Miraculously, his kidneys began to function again, and when they did, he no longer fit the Medicare eligibility criteria for hospice and he had to leave. In a book that he wrote during the final year of his life, he attested to the compassion and skill of the hospice caregivers and how they helped him to live his final days on his own terms (Buchwald, 2006).

While Buchwald's experiences with hospice are consistent with many hospice patients, there are others whose experiences are anything but positive. For example, when a family in Pennsylvania entered a hospice home care program, they were promised that nurses would be available around the clock to help them allow their loved one to die at home. When they called in the middle of the night in desperation for help when they were unable to control his pain and agitation during his final hours, they were told to take him to the emergency room. The nurse said that they weren't responsible for symptoms that were not related to his "terminal diagnosis." When another patient entered another hospice program, he begged to remain at home but was told that he would have to be admitted to their hospice facility because he was too sick. The real reason, as the family would learn, was that it was more cost-effective for the hospice to care for him on an inpatient basis. The sad truth is that these are not isolated cases, and increasingly, stories of "hospice horrors" and allegations of fraud and abuse are appearing in the popular media. Health services research reveals that over 30 years after hospice emerged as a humane terminal care reform, serious inadequacies in our model of end-of-life care remain (Robert Wood Johnson Foundation, 2002; SUPPORT Principal Investigators, 1995). But how and why have we arrived at this point? To begin to answer this question, it is helpful to explore the development of the American hospice movement and how the politics of health policy shaped it.

Setting the Stage for Terminal Care Reform

The experience of dying changed dramatically in the United States during the 20th century. Public health measures significantly decreased mortality rates during pregnancy, infancy, and childhood. Scientific and medical advances allowed patients to be clutched back from the hands of death and even promised renewal through organ transplantation. These advances were cause for celebration, but they did not at first reveal the impact longevity would have on the quality of life. The number of Americans living with chronic debilitating diseases increased significantly, and prolonged dying accompanied the longevity. By the end of the 1960s, cancer and complications of chronic disease caused over 60% of the deaths in the United States (Backer, Hannon, & Russell, 1982; Lerner, 1975).

During the 1960s, seminal research in sociology and nursing, funded primarily by the U.S. Public Health Service Division of Nursing, began to document the stark realities of institutionalized dying: pain control was virtually nonexistent, and many people died in a room at the end of the hall, behind a closed door, and alone (Glaser & Strauss, 1965, 1968; Quint, 1967; Sudnow, 1967). Too often, needless suffering often accompanied death for both the dying and the bereaved. Within the walls of medical centers, death was often considered by the medical establishment to be a mark of failure. Physicians rarely discussed terminal prognoses, maintaining that it was in the patient's best interests not to speak about it, and nurses and families joined the conspiracy of silence. The impact of this philosophy was significant. In one study, more than 50% of the hospitalized patients expressed fear and anxiety, often related to the response of physicians and nurses to their concerns. Patients reported overhearing nurses talking in the halls about other patients, often with graphic details about the horrors of disease. Patients who were not dying were very aware of patients who were. It was frightening for patients to listen to the sound of carts taking bodies away and hearing families crying (Duff & Hollingshead, 1968).

Additional research revealed that these conditions also had severe implications for staff on units where the death rate was high. One study conducted on a cancer ward observed that physicians and nurses considered the patients "walking dead," and patients constantly complained about "uncaring doctors," "unavailable nurses," and experimental drugs that they thought were being used on them as if they were guinea pigs (Death in a Cancer Ward, 1969, p. 56). Whereas at one time death was considered a natural occurrence, its medicalization transformed it into a distinctly unnatural event.

Hospice and the Call for Reform

In response to these conditions, reformers outside the walls of hospitals began to call for the reform of care provided within them. The civil and women's rights, death-with-dignity, and consumer movements were foundational to a growing public discourse about the quality of life, patients' rights, and the role of informed consent in the medical system. Stories of how terminal cancer patients suffered while undergoing experimental "rescue therapies" were widely disseminated in the popular press and left many Americans wondering whether the quest for cure was worth the human toll in suffering. In the case of hospice, idealistic reformers called for the release of dying patients from the social isolation of medical institutions and supported them as they returned home to the care of those most important to them. It was within this context that the hospice movement was born, and British physician Cicely Saunders would emerge as one of its charismatic leaders (Buck, 2005).

Hands Across the Waters: Conception of the Modern Hospice Movement

The modern hospice concept was first introduced to American health professionals in 1963 when British physician Cicely Saunders, the acknowledged founder of the modern hospice movement, made the first of many trips to North America (Clark, 1998, 2001, 2002; du Boulay, 1984; Seibold, 1992). During this first visit, Saunders spent 6 weeks traveling and lecturing about her work and research at St. Joseph's Hospice, a Catholic institution that was founded by the Irish Sisters of Charity in 1905 (Saunders, 1966). During these lectures, Saunders characterized St. Christopher's, the hospice she was building, as "a community...a common giving of people who share the cost of being vulnerable" (Saunders, 1971, p. 8). This philosophy of care broke down the artificial barriers between the physical, spiritual, and emotional aspects of care, and it blurred the boundaries of how health professionals and patients existed in relationship to each other. Her charismatic speaking style and passion for hospice care resonated with a small but growing cadre of idealistic health professionals who would put hospice forth as the antidote for institutionalized dying in America.

Saunders' first visit was a milestone in terminal care reform, and it also marked the beginning of a deep and lasting relationship between Saunders and Florence Wald, who is considered by many to be the American hospice midwife. When Wald first heard Saunders speak, she was Dean of the Yale School of Nursing and at a critical point in her life. A self-identified idealist, she had grown increasingly frustrated by the trend in medicine to focus on cure and technology rather than people. She firmly believed that nurses should be equal partners in care decisions as well as serving as leaders of interdisciplinary care teams (Wald, 1966). Given the era of broad social reform, Wald believed if she was ever going to make her mark on clinical nursing, the time was ripe. Saunders' conceptualization of hospice and the centrality of nursing within it offered the perfect vehicle by which she could achieve a "brave new world" in health care with nursing and medicine as equals at the helm (Foster & Corless, 1999; Wald, interview with author, December 19, 2000, New Haven, CT).

In 1966, Wald made a commitment to hospice, stepped down as dean, and brought together a group of like-minded individuals to research and reform care for the dying in the New Haven area. After a serendipitous meeting with Edward Dobihal and two other colleagues one afternoon, her plans to develop a "St. Christopher's in the Field" began to solidify. In 1968, Wald received funding from the U.S. Public Health Service Division of Nursing and the American Nurses Foundation to conduct the *Nurse's Study of the Terminally Ill Patient and His Family* and the subsequent *Interdisciplinary Study of the Dying Patient and His Family* (Wald, 1969). The studies served to coalesce and crystallize the group's vision for the creation of their own hospice, but they also offered a vehicle by which the group could work within a medical center to create individual and institutional change. In 1971, the group formalized operations as Hospice, Inc. and began serious planning to provide hospice care at home and in their own hospice facility (Dobihal, interview with author, July 11, 2002, Hamden, CT; Wald, interview, 2000). Despite their idealistic fervor and unwavering commitment to the hospice ideal, navigating the turbulent waters of the Connecticut medical system in an era of shifting political agendas for health care reform proved to be no small feat.

The Politics of Health Care Reform in the 1970s

Health care reform during the 1970s was multifaceted. By 1960, the many working Americans had some form of health insurance through their employers, but the vast majority of the 11.5 million American citizens age 62 or older did not (Social Security Administration, 2002). With a growing population of well-educated and politically powerful elders, considerable pressure was placed on politicians to pass legislation to assure that they, too, could have access to health care without losing everything they owned to pay for it. President Lyndon B. Johnson placed passage of Medicare and Medicaid on the top of his political agenda and won passage of the legislation in 1965.

Politicians did not fully anticipate the indirect economic impact of political concessions made to hospitals and physicians to assure passage of Medicare, but they were significant. Between 1963 and 1968, the costs of new programs administered by the Department of Health, Education, and Welfare grew dramatically. National health care spending rose from $100 billion to $168 billion, and the federal share of the bill rose from $32.6 billion to $61 billion. Due to the popularity of the Medicare program, Social Security spending jumped from $17 billion to $30 billion in 2 ½ years, an increase of approximately 75% (Scully, 2002). Between 1965 and 1970, national health expenditures rose from $41.7 billion to $74.7 billion; as a percentage of the gross national product (GNP), they rose from 6% to 7.5%. During those same years, the GNP expanded from $691 billion to $992.7 billion (Gibson, Waldo, & Levit, 1983). By the end of the Johnson administration, Medicare provided hospital insurance to 19.6 million people and supplemental insurance to 18.7 million (Social Security Administration). Per capita spending for health care had climbed to $357 and was 27% higher than any other country in the world. Legislators began to feel the financial impact of the Medicare legislation on the federal budget. Confronted with an escalating national deficit, a runaway health care industry, and the expansion of legislative responsibility for health care, Congress was compelled to find ways to hold costs down. One method of reform was to shift care away from the hospital and back into the home (Buhler-Wilkerson, 2001).

The expansion of public and private insurance during the latter half of the 20th century held promise for organizations providing home care, but it came at a cost. Until the advent of Medicare, Visiting Nurse Associations (VNAs) were the primary providers of home care in Connecticut and elsewhere (Buhler-Wilkerson, 2001; VNA of New Haven, 1977). Medicare reimbursement for home care impacted VNAs in several significant ways. First, the patient population shifted from mothers and babies to the elderly. In 1970, only 37.6% of all nursing visits at one VNA were illness focused; by 1980, 99.2% were (Daubert, 1981). During this era of deinstitutionalization, patients were being discharged from the hospitals quicker and sicker. The types of services and conditions under which these services would be reimbursable were defined not by patient need, but rather by strict Medicare eligibility criteria. For patients who met these criteria and had a need for "skilled nursing," Medicare would reimburse for up to 100 home care visits planned and "supervised" by the patient's physician (Buhler-Wilkerson, 2001). Surprisingly, physicians did not receive reimbursement for supervision. Unlike hospitals, VNAs were required to have Medicare certification, and the requisite paperwork and governmental oversight associated with reimbursement was extensive. As one VNA representative wrote in a 1967 annual report: "Medicare had added tremendously to the volume and complexity of our record keeping" (p. 1). In 1965, one person handled all of the reimbursement issues, but by 1967, 15 administrative staff members were dealing "exclusively with Medicare detail" (Rauch, 1967, p. 1).

Whereas VNAs realized the administrative challenges associated with these reforms, proprietary home care agencies saw the fiscal possibilities inherent in them. Reimbursement potential, combined with the demographics of a growing number of Medicare beneficiaries in need of home care, sweetened the pot. For-profit home care programs proliferated. Between 1966 and 1987, their number grew from 2,000 to over 10,000, and Medicare payments to them from $25 million to $4 billion (Gibson et al., 1983). Legislative efforts to expand social health insurance and then reform health care through privatization indirectly resulted in continued escalation of health care costs, increased oversight, and allegations of fraud. Wedged in the vice of health care reform, VNAs tried to balance social and medical needs of the patients and their families, while complying with federal and state mandates. In the words of one VNA administrator who wrote of the impact of these reforms:

> limited field staff, severely ill patients, endless audits by Medicare certifiers, constant meetings for interpretation...but by far the greatest burden to the staff was the pressure of the multiplication of competing agencies for the "paying" patient and the absolute absence of service for patients for whose care there was no source of payment. (Kauffman, 1974, p. 7)

The Impact of Policy on Practice

The hospice movement in Connecticut began in an era of cooperation between Hospice, Inc. and the local VNA. Unlike the VNAs who had to contend with the particulars and peculiarities of the formal reimbursement streams, Hospice Inc.'s home care program was funded through charitable contributions and grants from private foundations. Even when they received demonstration grant funding from the National Cancer Institute (NCI), they still had relative freedom to provide services attuned to the needs of individual patients and families. Still, many patients came into the program overwhelmed by bills accrued during prolonged illness. One patient's story reflected the experiences of many uninsured patients who were too rich for Medicaid and too young for Medicare. The patient was a 48-year-old, self-employed man. When he entered hospice, he was paying off $12,000 in hospital bills at $50.00 per month. The man could have qualified for Medicaid by disposing of his assets, but he would then have left his wife and three young children with nothing when he died (Lack & Buckingham, 1978). Hospice, Inc.'s home care team tried to help this man and his family but were frustrated by the fact that the vast resources available during the 1960s were drying up, and given the economic downturn of the 1970s, more and more people were in need.

The Hospice Entrepreneurs

By 1975, Hospice, Inc.'s home care program was growing rapidly. Notwithstanding the program's growth, financial concerns were omnipresent, the program's viability once the NCI demonstration project ended was in question, and there was considerable debate about how soon to integrate into the existing system of health care financing. Wald was adamant that they should follow Saunders's advice to "get it right," meaning the development of their model of hospice care prior to integrating into the system. Many on the board agreed with her to some degree, but it was clear to those with a more pragmatic approach that they needed formalized reimbursement streams sooner rather than later. Given the shifting political templates at the state and national level, it also was clear that they needed someone with the political savvy to help them navigate the turbulent waters of the Connecticut health care system. Dennis Rezendes fit the bill and was hired first as a consultant in 1973 and as a full-time executive director in 1974.

Under Rezendes's leadership, Hospice, Inc. went through a critical transition period, and, of necessity, new leadership styles emerged. The early development of Hospice, Inc. was fueled by the unfettered idealism of its early leaders. Whereas their enthusiasm served as a magnet to attract support for hospice, when they entered an environment in which utopian ideals and good intentions were not necessarily synonymous with organizational viability, they floundered. New leaders emerged, and those who were not able or willing to adapt to the requisite changes to move hospice forward were pushed to the periphery. By 1978, Wald was no longer affiliated with Hospice, Inc., and the entrepreneurial Dennis Rezendes was both creating and cornering the market for hospice at the state level.

Let the Political Games Begin: An Era of Cooptation

Over the next few years, Rezendes carved out a niche for hospice in an increasingly competitive health care marketplace. In 1976, he achieved a political victory for state legislation that liberalized Medicaid eligibility criteria for home care for terminally ill patients (Buck, 2005;

Lack & Buckingham, 1978). In 1978, he patented the term *hospice,* set strict criteria for its use, and secured legislation that designated hospice as a distinct type of health care provider *and* health care facility under Connecticut State Law. This legislation allowed Hospice, Inc., the only group that met its regulatory requirements, to capitalize on existing reimbursement for both home *and* institutional care for the dying. That same year, Rezendes joined forces with Don Gaetz and Hugh Westbrook, two hospice entrepreneurs from Florida, to form the National Hospice Organization (NHO; Beresford & Connor, 1999). Their mission was to both create and corner the market for hospice at the national level, and standardization of hospice was a critical element of their potential success. Although earlier definitions of hospice emphasized the importance of nursing and the family, NHO leaders were attentive to the need to define hospice in terms that would be politically palatable to legislators and influential special interest groups. Their guidelines reflected the necessity for hospice to conform to a medical-based policy. Within that context, nursing, social work and other professional services would be provided by an interdisciplinary team under the direction of a physician (NHO, 1981).

By 1978, the burgeoning hospice movement had created sufficient "noise" to gain the attention and support of many in Congress. While there was growing public support for hospice, one government study revealed the exponential growth in hospice programs across the country, with considerable variability in the configuration, type, and quality of services provided (Government Accounting Office [GAO], 1979). Further research was needed to test hospice's potential for nationalization. In 1978, a private–public partnership was created to support the 2-year National Hospice Study (NHS), which began in 1980, to substantiate whether or not hospice was superior to and more cost-effective than standard care for the dying (Aiken & Marx, 1982).

While the NHS study was underway, NHO leaders were busy crafting the Medicare hospice legislation and developing the requisite political support to assure its enactment. In a brilliant display of political maneuvering, Rezendes, Gaetz, and Westbrook gained the support of powerful congressional leaders, conservative and liberal. In 1980, Representative Leon Panetta introduced the hospice legislation in the House. When the legislation died in committee, Rezendes, Gaetz, and Westbrook launched a massive advocacy campaign. Their painstaking, grassroots efforts paid off in December 1981 when Panetta made good on his promise to reintroduce the legislation in the House of Representatives with 242 cosponsors (U.S. House of Representatives, 1982). Senator John Heinz (R-PA) introduced a companion bill in the Senate. Hospice had bipartisan and bicameral support, and the prospects looked hopeful.

Despite the momentum, they still faced an uphill battle during this era of retrenchment and reform. In setting his agenda in the 1982 State of the Union Address, President Ronald Reagan proclaimed: "Between 1972 and 1982, Medicare and Medicaid expenditures increased from $11.2 billion to almost $60 billion. Waste and fraud are serious problems...The time has come to control the uncontrollable" (1982). A conservative tone was set for the debates that ensued over the hospice legislation. Congressional testimony reveals that these debates were framed by four major constituencies: (1) the NHO, which supported the bill; (2) the home health industry, which opposed it; (3) legislators, who were divided on the issue for a variety of political and economic reasons; and (4) the Reagan Administration, which argued against it because of its desire to reform Medicare and the lack of conclusive cost data on hospice. These compelling and well-reasoned arguments against the hospice legislation notwithstanding, it passed in both the House and Senate by unanimous vote. In 1982, the Medicare hospice benefit became a reality with implementation scheduled for 1983 (Public Law 97–248, 1982). While preliminary data from the NHS was used to set the capitated reimbursement rate, otherwise the data was wholly ignored.

In the end, the NHS did not support hospice's claims (Mor, Greer, & Kastenbaum, 1988). Hospice was not found to be superior to standard institutional or home care in terms of quality of care. This finding might well attest to the effectiveness of hospice's educational efforts as well as shifting professional paradigms in nursing during this era. Hospice's cost-effectiveness was dependent upon patients with predictable death trajectories, cared for at home, with family caregivers and volunteers supplementing professional nursing care. While home hospice was more cost-effective than standard institutional care, it wasn't more cost-effective than traditional home care, primarily due to the increased number of professionals on interdisciplinary hospice teams (Oji-McNair, 1985). Nevertheless, in 1986, Congress elected to make the hospice benefit a permanent entitlement under Medicare and opened the door for reimbursement for hospice under Medicaid programs in 1986.

Given the lack of substantiating evidence to support hospice, why did they do this? The Congressional record reflects that they voted in favor of hospice for a variety of altruistic, political, and economic reasons. Legislators were swayed by compelling stories of dying patients and their families, their personal experiences with loss, and a *strong* message from constituents back home. They were also motivated by a deep concern about ever rising health care expenditures, the exponential growth of the hospice movement, and by a strong desire to control *it* before *it* controlled them. In a prelude to managed care, as the rules were promulgated, capitated payment rates were set for comprehensive core services, and although volunteer and bereavement services were mandated, reimbursement to cover the cost of providing these services was not incorporated in the rate. Eligibility criteria required that a patient be in the last 6 months of life, abandon all intensive treatment, and forfeit traditional Medicare benefits. In essence, this provision forced the patient to choose between curative treatment and death, left the physician with the difficult task of predicting exactly when that death would occur, and perhaps most vexing, telling the patient the truth.

While many within the hospice community celebrated passage of the legislation, still others were concerned about how it would shape hospice care. Their concerns were well founded. Today, hospice's reputation as a low-tech, high-touch integrative care for the mind, body, and spirit is gradually being supplanted by technologically driven and institutionally based care.

In conclusion, at the inception of the hospice movement, hospice was defined by the unfettered idealism of its founders. As the hospice concept was woven and rewoven into the fabric of the American medical system, new programs developed in accordance with the personal ideologies and professional paradigms of their founders and the environment in which they were created. Although they were all committed to a similar vision of what interdisciplinary hospice care should be, each group, each discipline, and, arguably, each individual viewed what this care entailed, where it should be provided, and who should be in control through slightly different social and cultural prisms. As the hospice became a legislated model of care, it was redefined by the politics of health policy and the health industry. Within this context, tensions between competing social, political, and economic factors created a paradoxical benefit that both decreased and increased barriers to care and ultimately served to further fragment, medicalize, and reinstitutionalize care for the dying. While many hospices remain true to their philosophical underpinnings and provide an invaluable service, still others are almost antithetical to its precepts and have come to resemble that which they were meant to reform.

PARTING WORDS ABOUT USING FRAMEWORKS

Frameworks provide historians with a structure to question and interpret historical data. In the case study presented, I began with the question of what happens to ideals about care as they are molded into legislated models of care. I used a social history framework to examine the grassroots beginnings of hospice and a policy framework to explicate how the politics of policy shaped the context of hospice as it was integrated into the system. Other frameworks, such as social, cultural, or even biographical, could have been used to ask other questions of the data. The frameworks that historians use, the questions that they ask, and the manner in which they analyze data are all influenced by the historian's interests, biases, background, and worldview. While historical frameworks help to guide inquiry, they are neither rigid nor static. Rather, as we see in the history of history, the relationship among frameworks, data, and the questions asked are reciprocal and dynamic, with each influencing the other. As for this historian, I look forward to seeing how these frameworks will be used and further refined by the future generations of nurse historians to come.

REFERENCES

Aiken, L., & Marx, M. (1982). Hospices: Perspectives on the public policy debate. *American Psychologist, 37*(11), 1271–1279.

Almond, G. A., & Verba, S. (1965). *The civic culture.* Boston: Little, Brown and Company.

Backer, B., Hannon, N., & Russell, N. (1982). *Death and dying: Individuals and institutions.* New York: Wiley.

Barzilai, G. (2003). *Communities and law: Politics and cultures of legal identities.* Ann Arbor: University of Michigan Press.

Beresford, L., & Connor, S. R. (1999). History of the National Hospice Organization. *Hospice Journal—Physical, Psychosocial, and Pastoral Care of the Dying, 14*(3–4), 15–31.

Braudel, F. (n.d.). *History quotes of a general nature.* American Society of Mechanical Engineers. Retrieved May 1, 2007, from http://www.asme.org/Communities/History/Resources/History_Quotes_General_Nature.cfm

Brush, B. (2002). Caring for life: Nursing during the Holocaust. *Nursing History Review, 10,* 69–81.

Brush, B. L., & Berger, A. M. (2002). Sending for nurses: Foreign nurse migration, 1965–2002. *Nursing and Health Policy Review, 1*(2), 103–115.

Brush, B. L., Sochalski, J., & Berger, A. M. (2004). Imported care: Recruiting foreign nurses to U.S. health care facilities. *Health Affairs, 23*(3), 78–87.

Buchwald, A. (2006). *Too soon to say goodbye.* New York: Random House.

Buck, J. (2004). Home hospice versus home health: Cooperation, competition, and co-optation. *Nursing History Review, 12,* 25–46.

Buck, J. (2005). Rights of passage: Reforming care for the dying, 1965–1986 (Doctoral Dissertation, University of Virginia, 2005). *Dissertation Abstracts International, 66*(03), 1389. (UMI No. AAT 3169641)

Buck, J. (2007). Reweaving a tapestry of care: Religion, nursing, and the meaning of hospice, 1945–1978. *Nursing History Review, 15,* 113–145.

Buhler-Wilkerson, K. (2001). *No place like home: A history of nursing and home care in the United States.* Baltimore: Johns Hopkins University Press.

Burke, P. (2004). *What is cultural history?* Cambridge, MA: Polity Press.

Clark, D. (1998). Originating a movement: Cicely Saunders and the development of St. Christopher's Hospice, 1957–1967. *Mortality, 3*(1), 43-53.

Clark, D. (2001). A special relationship: Cicely Saunders, the United States, and the early foundations of the modern hospice movement. *Illness, Crisis, and Loss, 9*(1), 15–31.

Clark, D. (2002). *Cicely Saunders: Founder of the hospice movement, selected letters 1959–1999.* London: Oxford University Press.

Connolly, C. A. (2004). Beyond social history: New approaches to understanding the state of and the state in nursing history. *Nursing History Review, 12,* 5–24.

Critchlow, D. (1993). A prognosis of policy history: Stunted: Or deceivingly vital? A brief reply to Hugh Davis Graham. *The Public Historian, 15*(4), 50–61.

Critchlow, D. (1998). Integrating social history and the state: Policy history through case studies. *The History Teacher, 31*(4), 459–466.

D'Antonio, P. (1999). Revisiting and rethinking the rewriting of nursing history. *Bulletin of the History of Nursing, 73*(2), 268–290.

D'Antonio, P. (2007). Conceptual and methodological issues in historical research. In S. B. Lewenson & E. K. Herrmann (Eds.), *Capturing nursing history: A guide to historical methods in research* (pp.11–23). New York: Springer Publishing.

Daubert, E. (1981). A position paper on strategic planning, August 1981, Visiting Nurses Association for South Central Connecticut Papers, Barbara Bates Center for the Study of the History of Nursing, University of Pennsylvania, box 7, folder 103, p. 12.

Death in a cancer ward. (1969, June 20). *Time Magazine,* 56. Retrieved from http://www.time.com/time/magazine/article/0,9171,844881-1,00.html

Diers, D. (2004). *Speaking of nursing: Narratives of practice, research, policy and the profession.* Boston: Jones and Bartlett.

du Boulay, S. (1984). *Cicely Saunders: The founder of the modern hospice movement.* London: Hodder and Stoughton.

Duff, R., & Hollingshead, A. (1968). *Sickness and society.* New York: Harper & Row.

Feldman, H. R., & Lewenson, S. B. (2000). *Nurses in the political arena: The public face of nursing.* New York: Springer Publishing Company.

Foster, Z., & Corless, I. (1999). Origins: An American perspective. *Hospice Journal—Physical, Psychosocial, and Pastoral Care of the Dying, 14,* 9–13.

Fox, D. (1993). *Power and illness: The failure and future of American health policy.* Berkeley: University of California Press.

Geertz, C. (1973). Thick description: Toward an interpretive theory of culture. In *The interpretation of cultures: Selected essays* (pp. 3–30). New York: Basic Books.

Gibson, R., Waldo, D., & Levit, K. (1983). National Health Expenditures, 1982. *Health Care Financing Review, 5*(1), 1–31.

Glaser, B., & Strauss, A. (1965). *Awareness of dying.* Chicago: Aldine Publishing Company.

Glaser, B., & Strauss, A. (1968). *Time for dying.* Chicago: Aldine Publishing Company.

Gordon, C. (2004). *Dead on arrival: The politics of health care in twentieth-century America.* Princeton NJ: Princeton University Press.

Gottschalk, M. (2000). *The shadow welfare state: Labor, business, and the politics of health care in the United States.* Ithaca, NY: Cornell University Press.

Government Accounting Office. (1979). *Report to the Congress of the United States: Hospice Care—A growing concept in the United States.* HRD-79–50. 3–6-1979.

Grossberg, M. (1979). A report on the Conference on the History of American Public Policy. *The Public Historian, 1*(2), 23–33.

Howell, M., & Prevenier, W. (2001). *From reliable sources: An introduction to historical methods.* Ithaca, NY: Cornell University Press.

Kauffman, M. (1974). *Executive director report, 1974.* Visiting Nurse Society of Philadelphia, Barbara Bates Center for the Study of the History of Nursing at the University of Pennsylvania, box 10, folder 93, p. 2.

Kertzer, D. I. (1996). *Politics and symbols.* New Haven, CT: Yale University Press.

Lack, S., & Buckingham, R. (1978). *First American hospice: Three years of home care.* New Haven, CT: Hospice, Inc.

Lerner, M. (1975). Where, why, and when people die. In O. G. Brim, H. E. Freeman, S. Levine, & N. A. Scotch (Eds.), *The dying patient.* New York: Russell Sage Foundation.

Lloyd, C. (1991). The methodologies of social history: A critical survey and defense of structurism. *History and Theory, 30*(2), 180–219.

Lukacs, J. (2002). *At the end of an age.* Chicago: R. R. Donnelley & Sons.

Lynaugh, J. (2006). Mildred Tuttle: Private initiative and public response in nursing education after World War II. *Nursing History Review, 14,* 203–211.

Marmor, T. (2000). *The politics of medicare* (2nd ed.). New York: Aldine De Gruyter.

Mechanic, D., & Reinhard, S. (2002). Contributions of nurses to health policy: Challenges and opportunities. *Nursing and Health Policy Review, 1*(1), 7–15.

Mor, V., Greer, D., & Kastenbaum, R. (1988). *The hospice experiment.* Baltimore MD: The Johns Hopkins University Press.

National Hospice Organization. (1981). *Standards of a hospice program of care.* McLean, VA: Author.

Neustadt, R., & May, E. (1986). *Thinking in time: The uses of history for decision makers.* New York: The Free Press.

Novick, P. (1988). *That noble dream: The objectivity question and the American historical profession.* New York: Cambridge University Press.

Oberlander, J. (2003). *The political life of medicare.* Chicago: University of Chicago Press.

Oji-McNair, K. (1985). The cost analysis of hospice versus non-hospice care: Positioning characteristics for marketing a hospice. *Health Marketing Quarterly,* 2(4), 119–129.

Oliver, T. (2004, August). Policy entrepreneurship in the social transformation of American medicine: The rise of managed care and managed competition. *Journal of Health Politics, Policy and Law, 29,* 701–733.

Oliver, T., Lee, P., & Lipton, H. (2004, June). A history of medicare and prescription drug coverage. *Milbank Quarterly, 82,* 283–354.

Public Law 97–248. (1982). Retrieved from http://www.ssa.gov/OP_Home/comp2/F097-248.html

Quint, J. (1967). *The nurse and the dying patient.* New York: The Macmillan Company.

Rauch, F. (1967). *Annual report of the President, 2 November 1967.* Visiting Nurses Society of Philadelphia, Center for the Study of the History of Nursing, School of Nursing, University of Pennsylvania, series I, box 5, folder 86, p. 1.

Reagan, R. (1982). *1982 State of the Union Address.* Retrieved June 13, 2007, from http://65.126.3.86/reagan/html/reagan_speeches.shtml

Robert Wood Johnson Foundation. (2002). *Last acts: Means to a better end: A report on dying in America today.* Washington, DC: Last Acts National Program.

Sampson, D. (2006). *Determinants and determination: Negotiating nurse practitioner prescribing legislation in New Hampshire, 1973–1985.* Unpublished doctoral dissertation, University of Pennsylvania, Philadelphia.

Saunders, C. (1966). *The moment of truth.* Unpublished paper presented at Yale University, May, 1966. Dame Cicely Saunders Papers, Hospice History Project, Sheffield, England, box 57, 2/1/92, p. 1.

Saunders, C. (1971). The patient's response to treatment: A photographic presentation. *Proceedings of the Fourth National Symposium, Catastrophic Illness in the Seventies: Critical Issues and Complex Decisions.* New York: Cancer Care, Incorporated.

Scully, G. (2000, July). *Public spending and social progress* (NCPA Policy Report 232). Dallas, TX: National Center for Policy Analysis. Retrieved from http://www.ncpa.org/~ncpa/studies/s232/s232.html

Seibold, C. (1992). *The hospice movement: Easing death's pains.* New York: Twayne Publishers.

Social Security Administration. *History of SSA during the Johnson Administration, 1963–1968.* Retrieved June 12, 2002, from http://www.ssa.gov/history/ssa/lbjleg1.html

Starr, P. (1982). *The social transformation of American medicine.* New York: Basic Books.

Stearns, P. (1983). Social and political history. *Journal of Social History, 16*(3), 3–5.

Stearns, P., & Tarr, J. (1993). Straightening the policy history tree. *The Public Historian, 15*(4), 63–67.

Stevens, R., Rosenberg, C., & Burns, L. (Eds.). (2006). *History and health policy: Putting the past back in.* New Brunswick, NJ: Rutgers University Press.

Sudnow, D. (1967). *Passing on: The social organization of dying.* Upper Saddle River, NJ: Prentice-Hall.

SUPPORT Principal Investigators. (1995). A controlled trial to improve care for seriously ill hospitalized patients: The study to understand prognoses and preferences for outcomes and risks of treatment (SUPPORT). *Journal of the American Medical Association, 274*(20), 1591–1599.

U.S. House of Representatives. (1982, March 25). *Coverage of hospice care under the Medicare program.* Washington, DC: House of Representatives, Committee on Ways and Means, Subcommittee on Health.

Visiting Nurse Association of New Haven, Inc. (1977, June 23). *Formal Evaluation Program, 1976–1977.* Visiting Nurse Association of South Central Connecticut, Center for the Study of the History of Nursing, School of Nursing, University of Pennsylvania, series I, box 3, folder 36, p. 3.

Wald, F. (1966). Emerging nursing practice. *American Journal of Public Health, 56*(8), 1252–1260.

Wald, F. (1970). Development of an interdisciplinary team to care for dying patients and their families. In *ANA Clinical Conferences, American Nurses Association, 1969, Minneapolis/Atlanta* (pp. 47–55). New York: Appleton-Century-Crofts.

Weissert, C., & Weissert, W. (2002). The policy process. In C. Weissert & W. Weissert (Eds.), *Governing health: The politics of health policy* (2nd ed., pp. 245–280). Baltimore, MD: Johns Hopkins University Press.

Wing, K. (2000). Health care reform in the year 2000: The view from the front of the classroom. *American Journal of Law and Medicine, 26,* 277–293.

Zelizer, J. (2000). Clio's lost tribe: Public policy history since 1978. *Journal of Policy History, 12*(3), 370–394.

Zelizer, J. (2005). Introductions: New directions in policy history. *Journal of Policy History, 17*(1), 1–11.

CHAPTER FIVE

Critical Issues in the Use of Biographic Methods in Nursing History

Sonya J. Grypma

bio: life graph: writing[1]

I brushed up against the renowned Canadian nurse Ethel Johns in front of a stone hearth in the Woodward Biomedical Library at the University of British Columbia. That is to say, I ran my fingertips along the edges of her aged letters, mostly typed on blue tissue-thin paper with a jumpy typewriter. I had already read Margaret Street's comprehensive, award-winning biography and through it became acquainted with Johns and her unique brand of nursing leadership during the 1920s and 1930s.[2] Street did not have access to the letters I fingered, however, and handling them brought a thrill of discovery. I began to comprehend the allure of historiography. However, nursing historiography is undergoing change, and the relevance of the biographic method is being challenged. Historians of nursing are promoting a "new historiography": Patricia D'Antonio is urging scholars to "revisit and rethink the rewriting of nursing history"; Christopher Maggs is calling for a "new approach to defining historical

Acknowledgments: The author wishes to thank Janet Ross Kerr, Pauline Paul, and Margaret Haughey of the University of Alberta for their feedback and support. Thanks also to NHR's anonymous reviewers. This project was funded in part by the Social Sciences and Humanities Research Council of Canada, the Walter Izaak Killam Memorial Trust, and Dr. Shirley Stinson.

questions and a new search for meanings"; Sioban Nelson is asking historians to reconsider the purpose and audience of nursing history.[3] The new historiography rejects nursing's "cosy profession-centred celebration of its past," emphasizing issues or themes such as ethics, technology, civics, and religion rather than focusing on nursing's "great women."[4] If the biographic method is to remain relevant in the new nonsubject-centered milieu, biography must be approached and written in new ways. After a brief argument in favor of the biographic method, the present chapter revisits and revises methodological concerns raised by others, focusing on four critical issues in the use of biographic methods in nursing history: selecting a "worthy" subject, dealing with limited sources, exemplifying truth in data analysis, and writing a compelling report.

RELEVANCE OF THE BIOGRAPHIC METHOD

Nursing is a rich and virtually untapped international field from which to choose subjects for a biographical study. While recognizing the universality of biographic methods in nursing, this chapter focuses on examples from Canadian nursing history. Nurses have made up the largest professional workforce in Canada, and Canadian nursing history extends back three and a half centuries.[5] Yet the number of biographic studies of Canadian nurses remains surprisingly small. In 1975, the year Margaret Street wrote her biography of Ethel Johns, there existed almost no biographic studies of outstanding members of the profession in Canada.[6] In the three decades since then, historical studies of varying depth have been conducted on Canadian nurse leaders Edith Kathleen Russell, Jean I. Gunn, Elizabeth McMaster, and Caroline Wellwood, among others.[7] Reasons for the paucity of biographic studies may include the low status of biography within the discipline of history, the low status of historical research within the discipline of nursing, and the low status of nurses within society.[8] Janet Ross Kerr notes that nursing has always been susceptible to biases associated with gender as the nursing workforce has been primarily composed of women.[9] Thus, the lack of scholarly interest in nurses may be partly related to the historic lack of interest in women. However, even scholars interested in nursing and in women are not choosing biographic methods: only two of nineteen doctoral studies listed in the "New Dissertations" section of the 2003 volume of *Nursing History Review* were biographies.[10] As nursing historiography moves toward an emphasis on themes rather than individuals, the biography risks becoming obsolete.[11] Despite waning scholarly interest in biographic methods (or perhaps because of it) there is a growing need for biographic studies—particularly of ordinary nurses' lives. For purposes of this chapter, the term "*biographic method*" is used to describe any historiographical approach that seeks to understand the life of an individual person; "*nursing biographies*" refers to studies of the professional lives of individual nurses.

A decade ago the emphasis of biography was on "great women." M. Louise Fitzpatrick identified the need for studies of "Great Persons," and Natalie Riegler identified a need for women's stories.[12] Today, Sioban Nelson asks, "What does nursing history begin to look like *minus* its great women?"[13] This rhetorical question signals a change of direction in historiography and corresponds with new opportunities for biographers. For example, as academic interest shifts toward the lives of ordinary people,[14] space is created for biographic studies of both male and female nurses in a range of professional roles. Also, as the function of historiography shifts from edification of members of the nursing profession to increasing the visibility of nursing history among the general public,[15] biography's ongoing popularity in bookstores and potential to hold a reader's interest in the larger subject may increase its appeal for researchers. If the biographic method is to remain relevant in nursing historiography, one critical issue to be addressed is the selection of "*worthy*" nurses.

ADDRESSING WORTHINESS IN SUBJECT SELECTION

The initial response to the uneasy question of who is "*worthy*" of a biographic study may be to identify nursing's elite—those who are praiseworthy and admirable. If the purpose of nursing biography is understood as providing prototypes for the development of leaders,[16] the focus naturally turns to those who held positions of leadership in institutional hierarchies or played key roles in historical milestones. Indeed, all the subjects of the Canadian biographies mentioned above were administrators at some point in their careers. Jean Gunn, Ethel Johns, and Kathleen Russell were intelligent, determined, and politically astute leaders in interwar Canada who made remarkable and significant contributions to early nursing education at a time when patriarchal structures devalued the contribution of women. Whereas it is appropriate to herald the accomplishments of nursing leaders, a balanced portrait of nursing history should also include their disappointments and failures, as well as the experiences of "ordinary" nurses. If the purpose of nursing biography is revisioned to include "restoring to their rightful place [nurses] who have been ignored, misunderstood or forgotten" or "correcting distortions" of famous nurses,[17] a wider range of possibilities for biographic study is uncovered.

Selection of a subject for biographic research, then, is not limited to the traditional focus on public figures. As historiography moves from an "era of heroic biography to an era more interested in the archeology of humbler lives," work on the ordinary daily lives of subjects is increasingly possible and desirable.[18] This shift allows historians to work on the "lives of unknown or lesser known figures, exploring what their experience can offer to our understanding of an era, a movement, or a culture."[19] As with any scholarly research, selection of a subject—whether "great" or "ordinary"—should be considered carefully and in light of its value as a contribution to a field.[20] In 1914 Sir Edward Cook, biographer of Florence Nightingale, suggested that the subject of biography should have a memorable life and a distinctive and interesting character.[21] Scholarly interest in a person is not only as an individual human being, but also as a focal point within nursing history—and a relatively unique one.[22] Many possibilities exist in Canadian nursing. What would nursing history look like, for example, if we brought to light the life of an early graduate of the nursing program at the University of Toronto, who sipped tea at Kathleen Russell's gracious nursing residence and then went to the hospital wards to face the gritty world of illness and injury care? Or a male nurse who worked in the early gendered world of nursing in Vancouver? What of a Catholic Sister who left the dominant culture of Montreal in the 1930s to join other nursing nuns in St. Therese Hospital in Nunavut, Northern Canada? A Chinese student who completed her nurse's training in Lamont, Alberta, and then returned to war-torn China in the 1940s? A nurse in Lethbridge, Alberta, who converted her home into an isolation hospital during the Spanish Flu outbreak in 1918? Clearly there are many untold lives worth telling. By focusing on the lives of a variety of nurses engaged in a range of nursing responsibilities, scholars not only have the opportunity to acknowledge individual contributions to the profession, but also to examine the more subtle aspects of the relationships among nursing and gender, race, religion, civics, technology, community, and health.

In addition to illuminating the lives of previously unknown nurses, scholars may revisit the lives of famous ones, reinterpreting data through different lenses. The plethora of scholarship on Florence Nightingale—exploring everything from sanitary reforms to mysticism to lesbianism—attests to the variety of interpretations a single life may stimulate. Recently I've revisited aspects of Canadian nurse leader Ethel Johns's life in light of evidence unavailable to her biographer in 1975, including previously sealed records from the Rockefeller Foundation archives and correspondence between Johns and Kathleen Russell during the 1920s and 1930s.[23] This new evidence suggests that Johns was committed to racial equity during an era when such commitment was not the cultural norm, giving new significance to her upbringing on an Ojibwa reservation, her attraction to international fieldwork with the Rockefeller Foundation, and her ongoing attention to intercultural themes as editor of *Canadian Nurse*. As Elspeth Cameron has noted, two people with access to the same material would produce different versions of the same life.[24] Thus, any existing biography is open to reinterpretation.

When one assesses subject worthiness, intrigue is an often underrated consideration. The subject must hold particular appeal for the researcher, who should be able to transmit that sense of fascination to the reader. Intrigue keeps the researcher engaged through the more tedious aspects of the research process and holds the reader's attention and interest in the eventual research "product." Canadian nurse Jean Ewen is an example of an intriguing subject. Ewen wrote a candid and witty reminiscence of her years in China between 1932 and 1938, first as an inadvertent Catholic missionary nurse, and then under the auspices of the China Aid Council as an assistant to Dr. Norman Bethune.[25] Ewen vividly recalls her misadventures with the eccentric Bethune while traveling to Mao Ze-dong's Eighth Route Army camp deep in China's interior. She describes her frustration with Bethune (from whom she eventually parted) and her subsequent year of wandering alongside Chinese refugees and Red Army soldiers, narrowly avoiding Japanese bombing raids. A biography of Ewen is appealing for a number of reasons. First, she is virtually invisible in the major studies of the "martyred Norman Bethune."[26] Second, her autobiography contains several inconsistencies and gaps. For example, Ewen refers to an article in the *Chicago Tribune* "dated March 12, 1938... [which] said we were dead and ran Bethune's picture," but no such article exists.[27] Third, there are conflicting reports of the circumstances surrounding her departure from Bethune. Ewen suggests that Bethune conspired to get rid of her, but there is evidence that she left without notifying him, leaving him vexed about her whereabouts for months.[28] Finally, Ewen was a spirited participant in extraordinary events, and yet historians have treated her as little more than a source of information on Bethune. Ewen is a "worthy" subject for a biographic study. However, even such a suitable subject is impossible to research without access to sufficient sources.

ADDRESSING LIMITED SOURCES IN DATA COLLECTION

Access to sufficient sources is vital. Early in a study, the question of availability and location of primary sources must be addressed.[29] It is risky to undertake an in-depth study of a person's life without confirmed access to primary sources such as personal documents and firsthand accounts by those who knew the subject during the era under review. Without access to high quality material, the researcher will be frustrated, and the study's credibility will be undermined. The danger of forging ahead without sufficient resources is illustrated by a recent biography by Margaret Negodaeff-Tomsik titled *Honour Due: The Story of Dr. Leonora Howard King.*[30] Negodaeff-Tomsik started her investigation of Howard after reading an obscure bibliographical paragraph about her in a turn-of-the-century *Who's Who.* Negodaeff-Tomsik was intrigued and undertook her study despite few primary sources (most of Howard's letters were lost in the 1960s, and no diaries were found). Her subsequent overreliance on secondary sources is problematic, turning a potential scholarly work into a "fictionalized biography: factual gaps filled in with a novelist's imagination."[31] A brief critique of Negodaeff-Tomsik's study will underscore the importance of primary sources and broad historical knowledge of the subject's social, cultural, and political context—a point I return to later.

Leonora Howard King was the first Canadian physician in China (1877–1925) and the first Western woman to be made a Mandarin. Compared with the lives of other women in Canada, Howard's experience was certainly extraordinary. Compared with the lives of other Canadian missionaries in China, however, it was not exceptional, despite Negodaeff-Tomsik's claims to the contrary. Three examples illustrate how using decontextualized quotes from secondary sources can raise concerns about a study's credibility. First, Negodaeff-Tomsik declares that Roman Catholic missions did not venture into the field of modern medicine, noting that the extent of medical service by the Grey Sisters from Pembroke, Ontario, was "handing out quinine tablets and worm pills" to the Chinese.[32] This comment, though not referenced, is clearly excerpted from a paragraph in Alvyn Austin's *Saving China* and overlooks the significance of the Grey Sisters, who, as early nurse practitioners, diagnosed and treated thousands of patients in China suffering from a comprehensive range of illness and injury.[33] Second, Negodaeff-Tomsik notes that Canadian evangelist Jonathan Goforth believed in Divine Healing, another unreferenced quote, this time from Stursberg's *Golden Hope.*[34] From this she surmises that Goforth would have opposed Howard's medical practice (which included cataract surgery), but she overlooks the fact that the earliest medical missionaries in Goforth's station of North Honan performed cataract surgery and that Goforth himself underwent eye surgery.[35] Finally, Negodaeff-Tomsik quotes Canadian physician Robert McClure's description of the early days of medicine to contrast with Howard's work (another unreferenced quote from *Saving China*).[36] However, McClure's work in North Honan did not begin until 1924, a few months before Howard's death: It was Robert's father, William McClure, who would have been Howard's contemporary.[37]

Absence of personal documents does not automatically preclude a biographical study, provided other high quality primary sources are available. Natalie Kegler notes that, even in the absence of personal chapters, she managed to get at the truth about Canadian nurse Jean Gunn through labor-intensive research in libraries and archives, information from journals, interviews with Gunn's students, and hospital and nursing reports.[38] Kegler measured evidence sufficiency in terms of whether it allowed the subject to remain in the foreground. When there is insufficient evidence, the subject becomes lost in the background of events, actions, and circumstances, making it difficult to acquaint readers with the subject's personhood—how he or she responded to events rather than just the events themselves.

Metaphors abound in references describing the nature of historical data collection. Biographers become "detectives" and "archaeologists who "mine" and "dig" for sources, "leaving no stone unturned" as they work to "piece together" the "puzzles" of a "buried life. The serendipity of unexpected discovery often fuels the search.[39] After a subject is chosen, the search for sources usually starts in libraries and archives. Documents on topics such as the subject's career, family, education, and relationships may include records, minutes from meetings, newspaper clippings, and alumnae records. Friends and family of the subject sought via organization advertisements (e.g., church or nursing alumnae publications) may provide personal chapters such as diaries, journals, and photos. As the stack of evidence grows, the need for a broad understanding of the historical context becomes clearer: a well-prepared researcher can separate high-quality sources from mounds of minutiae by approaching sources with questions, and the best questions are developed with an understanding of existing historical scholarship of the period and profession under study. According to Kathleen Cruikshank, if the right questions are asked, "the mountains of trivia will melt away and essences will emerge."[40] Questions should be continually revised and expanded as the research continues, aiming to "struggle to answer all the questions that the accessible materials provoke." In the study of human history, eyewitness accounts of events are of key importance.[41] Historians necessarily rely on the observations of others to piece together an understanding of the character of a subject, or of a particular change over time. Yet relying on others' observations restricts the historical researcher to what these observers believe they believe or what they are willing to reveal.[42]

To get around the problem of limited perspectives, the historian must collect various views of the same event. For this reason, a study should involve at least four views. First, an overview (birds-eye view) of relevant sociopolitical events in the historical period under study can be sought through existing historical scholarship. Second, firsthand accounts (ground view) of persons living through the period can be sought through data recorded during the period, such as newschapter articles, reports, and letters. Especially compelling are documents such as diaries and confidential files, as these are less mediated than official reports by secretaries or journalists. As Marc Bloch noted in 1941, "Who among us would not prefer to get hold of a few secret chancellery chapters or some confidential military reports, to having all the newschapters of 1938 or 1939?"[43] We are eagerly drawn to that which we were not intended to overhear. Third, recollections of experiences after the period under study has passed (rear view) can be sought through oral interviews, autobiographies, and memoirs. Whereas the ground view contains raw data, the rear view contains processed data—it has been interpreted over time. Finally, an understanding of the values, beliefs, and assumptions of subjects (worldview) may be sought through reading between the lines of first-person accounts and reminiscences. Personal recollections may reveal as much about the author's worldview as they do about sociopolitical events.

There is debate among historians regarding the value of recollections in general, and the use of data from oral interviews in particular. According to M. Louise Fitzpatrick, oral interviews may be used to corroborate and clarify written material, help connect disparate pieces of information, and assist with the interpretation of patterns of events. However, they may also be unreliable because of their tendency to be colored by egocentrism, hyperbole, and selective memory.[44] Fitzpatrick suggests that interviews be completed only after data have been collected from documents.

Alice Wexler is less skeptical of oral interviews, suggesting that reminiscences are valuable provided the researcher is clear about the distinction between the memory of a life and a life actually lived. To Wexler, recollections represent a person's construction of self and give insight into the ongoing tension among people's sexual, racial, economic, and cultural selves.[45] Recollections should be approached with the understanding that they reflect a particular worldview and may represent a particular agenda—but so should other sources of data. According to Dee Garrison all writers bring their particular values and beliefs to their writing consciously or not.[46] Therefore, all evidence should be analyzed in terms of the motives and social positions of the authors.[47] According to Sioban Nelson, the challenge for contemporary researchers is to understand the perspective of the authors of sources and the context in which those sources were produced.[48] Apparently getting at the "truth" of a subject involves more than meets the eye.

ADDRESSING "TRUTH" IN DATA ANALYSIS

Fitzpatrick contends that the purpose of historiography in nursing is to discover truth.[49] Because an ontological debate about the existence of truth and the nature of reality is beyond the scope of this chapter, the term "*truth*" will be used here to refer to the accuracy and reliability of the study. That is, the challenge of the biographer is to produce a true (or accurate) portrait of a nursing subject. Finding the "image under the carpet"[50] goes beyond subjects' self-perception and how others perceived them to how the subjects affected and were affected by a particular sociopolitical era. In attempting to produce a true portrait, the biographer is caught between the need to adhere to facts and the need to interpret a subject.[51] The biographic method involves more than a recital of facts, more than a description of the individual's minute doings, and more than a study of achievements.[52] At one extreme, accumulated facts can smother the subject.[53] At the other, interpretation with little evidence is unreliable. The difficulty of producing a truthful portrait of a subject is exemplified by the 1952 classic *The Scalpel, the Sword: The Story of Doctor Norman Bethune,* by Sydney Gordon and Ted Allan.

In their biography, Gordon and Allan pay homage to Bethune, who died of an infected scalpel nick incurred while operating on wounded soldiers at the front line of the Eighth Route Army in China in 1939. In China for less than 2 years, Bethune was adored by the Chinese for his surgical skill and selfless devotion to the army's wounded under the most extreme wartime conditions. His death secured his reputation as a hero and even a "saint." Written more like a novel than a historical document, *The Scalpel, the Sword* is an engaging account of Bethune's career. The writing style is remarkably similar to Bethune's own: artistic, reflective, and vivid. Although the authors quote frequently from Bethune's writing, they are liberal in their own interpretation of events. The lack of any referencing, combined with an eloquent writing style that matches Bethune's, makes it virtually impossible to separate fact from embellishment; Gordon and Allan's words flow seamlessly from Bethune's.

Their themes overlap with Bethune's, too. Gordon and Allan esteem the working people and those with the high moral ideals of socialism and Communism, disparaging both the Nationalists and missionaries, who purportedly did not similarly devote their lives to the cause.[54] Their suggestion that Bethune was the main, if not the only, physician helping the Chinese is odd, considering the number of medical missionaries in China, most notably Canadian physician Robert McClure, whom Bethune actually met.[55] It seems likely that Gordon and Allan served a political agenda in portraying Bethune as a singular Marxist humanitarian (as opposed to many Canadian medical personnel in China, mostly Christian missionaries). If their aim had been nonpartisan, it is improbable that they would have excluded Canadian nurse Jean Ewen, minimized the work of Bethune's partner, Richard Brown, and misrepresented Bethune's team as American rather than Canadian.[56] Mao Ze-dong's homage to Bethune shortly after his death may have secured his place in Chinese consciousness, but Gordon and Allan's portrayal of Bethune established his international reputation as a Communist hero.

The Scalpel, the Sword is a literary masterpiece. But does it portray truth? It certainly has been treated as truth—virtually every book or film portrayal of Bethune since 1952 draws largely from Gordon and Allan's work. Ken Mitchell, a professor of literature and one of Bethune's numerous biographers, wrote that to reach the heart of biographical truth, one must "rely less on the dictates of historical accuracy and documentary truth and more on a comprehension of character."[57] But how much of Gordon and Allan's own ideology and agenda shaped their portrayal of Bethune? Truth in biography is mediated, and most biographers tend to exaggerate the role of the protagonist while diminishing the supporting cast.[58] However, whereas a novelist may consciously create a symbolic persona, a scholar may not preconceive a subject's character, nor may a scholar ignore unexpected, unflattering, or damaging evidence.

According to Elspeth Cameron, truth in biography comes as a result of long-term immersion both in the available materials and in the personality of a subject. Over time, patterns emerge—patterns more valid if not preconceived by the biographer.[59] Biographers go about immersing themselves in their subjects' lives in different ways. Mitchell immersed himself in Norman Bethune's character by portraying Bethune in a one-person drama. He concluded that his creative interpretation was more truthful than "the photographic and documentary memorabilia of archival documents."[60] Dee Garrison spent 5 months living in the former home of Mary Heaton Vorse.[61] Kathryn Kish Sklar became so emotionally absorbed with Florence Kelly that she experienced a kinesthetic paralysis during the most intense phase of her study.[62] According to Alice Wexler, getting to know a subject takes a decade or two.[63] Though scholars' approaches may differ, their collective aim is to know their subjects as real and complex individuals.

Admiration for a particular subject may initiate researcher interest, but it should not preclude honesty. Riegler describes credibility in biography as being honest to oneself, the subject, and the reader.[64] Over the course of time, as the researcher becomes more intimately acquainted with the subject, a relationship of sorts forms, and the researcher may vacillate between admiration, rejection, and even dislike of the subject.[65] In the latter case, honesty may become more difficult. Jacquelyn Dowd Hall describes her concern with discrediting an admirable woman after finding unwelcome evidence.[66] She struggled with her own feelings of disappointment and dislike of her subject. She realized, however, that to ignore unflattering evidence would be to ignore truth. A biographer can be imaginative, but must not imagine the materials.[67]

As historians have "moved beyond examining only the successes of our past"[68] over the past decade or more, it has become possible to portray subjects as complex human beings who struggle, make mistakes, and may be unlikable. The complex interaction between nurses' private and public lives has assumed increasing importance to historians, and sensitivity to the "almost seamless interconnectedness of women's working and private lives" is considered essential.[69] Patricia D'Antonio notes that women's culture and experiences can never be completely understood just in terms of their relationship with paid labor, and that understanding women's places within the social fabric of their communities, neighborhoods, and families is key to understanding their consciousness, role, and agency.[70] She asks scholars of nursing to consider ways to reconcile the tendency to focus only on professional aspects of nurses' lives, with the knowledge that women rarely secured their identities solely in relation to productive employment. The biographic method is well suited to this type of exploration because biographers emphasize the importance of exploring personal lives and their impact on public accomplishment and aim to understand how private experiences shape public choices.[71] Feminist biographers in particular have been sensitive to gender-specific ways in which women have had to prove themselves both in the public and private sphere.[72] For historians of nursing, biographic studies hold great promise in helping to understand how nursing identity extended beyond the bounds of paid employment, because biography allows historians to position *identity* rather than *work* at the center of analyses.[73]

A final consideration when addressing truth in data analysis is attention to the historical context. According to Kathleen Cruikshank, without context there can be no interpretation or themes, for there are no reference points from which to draw them.[74] Understanding context involves understanding what was happening within the profession during a particular era, but also what was happening in the community at large. In writing about the history of education, Cruikshank contends that it is not possible to understand the life and work of a professional without the context of the history of the profession. Nor is it possible to regard a life and work as significant for professional history if it is not taken in that context. Similarly, historians of nursing require a good grasp of the profession's history. Historical data are rendered meaningful only through the analysis of a broader historical context.[75] Thus, in order to get at the truth of a nurse's life, careful attention must also be paid to issues such as economy, gender, race, national identity, social politics, militarism, and the history of medicine—that is, the context within which the nurse lived.[76]

WRITING A COMPELLING REPORT

If the new historiography aims to bring nursing to the broader community of historical scholars as well as to the general public, then research that is "rigorous, sophisticated and compelling will be best received.[77] The greatest asset of the biographic method is its ability to encompass the universal and the particular and hold the reader's interest in the larger subject.[78] Biography's emphasis on literary style is no doubt responsible for its popularity among readers. According to Francess Halpenny, biographic studies range from the most-literary/least-factual to the most-factual/least-literary, with the novel as biography at one end of the spectrum and compilation of sources at the other.[79] The most literary end is exemplified by Negodaeff-Tomsik's skillful but inaccurate biography. The most factual is exemplified by biographers who simply abridge a "chronological trek" through diary volumes.[80] Nursing scholarship should avoid either extreme, aiming instead for "literary grace" plus "a nourishment of insight on rigorous research."[81] One can easily underestimate the art of biography.[82] Compelling biography involves similar characteristics as compelling fiction, including antagonists (to contrast with the subject-as-protagonist), a central tension around which to organize the material, and development of believable characters and dramatization of crucial moments—all without conscious distortion of fact.[83] The following five recommendations may assist would-be biographers. First, writers must guide the reader, organizing the material in such away that the reader is left with a dominant impression, some major theme with which subsidiary themes resonate.[84] Second, length is not as important as quality. Most academic biographies are 400–500-page volumes, but there is also a need for shorter studies. Novice researchers may be less intimidated by a profile study than by a full-fledged biography, and the general public may be more inclined to read smaller publications. Third, writers should be explicit about their assumptions, distinguishing their own voice from that of their subjects. Riegler recommends letting the subject speak through the liberal use of quotes.[85] Fourth, writing should bring the subject to life. To Lynaugh, the "task of writing is to make the narrative live for the reader in the same way it thrills us as we discover it."[86] Finally, the writer should add scrupulous footnoting.[87] This not only gives credit to sources; it also allows readers to judge the breadth and depth of the research, follow the scholar's methodological trail, and verify interpretations. First-rate biography is carefully researched and skillfully written.

CONCLUSION

The new historiography calls for a new approach to defining historical questions and a search for new meanings. This chapter has revisited the biographical method to determine where revisions could strengthen its ability to meet contemporary challenges. To this end, four critical issues in the use of the biographical method in nursing history are highlighted. First, there is a need for a wider range of subjects. Researching nurses who represent a variety of roles and settings offers a broader range of questions and provides the opportunity to explore relationships between nursing and issues related to gender, race, religion, civics, technology, community, and health. Second, there is a need for careful attention to the quality of sources in data collection. Although lack of personal documents does not preclude a biographic study, accessible material should be rich enough to be probed deeply for meanings. Whether dealing with documents written during the period under study or with recollections, researchers must pay attention to the social context in which the documents were written and to the worldview of the author, taking notice of gaps and silences. Sources should be approached with questions generated by, and grounded in, formal study of the history of the period and of the nursing profession. Third, painting a truthful portrait of a subject involves immersion in the nurse's life, acceptance of unexpected or unflattering evidence, and willingness to let themes emerge from the data rather than preconceiving or imposing them. Finally, biographies must be compelling, scrupulously footnoted, and suited to a broad audience. Literary skill must be used to engage the reader while adhering to the facts; neither compilations of source materials nor fictional narratives are appropriate. Done well, the biographic method promises to be not only relevant, but to be on the cutting edge of nursing historical scholarship.

NOTES

1. T. F. Hoad, ed., *Concise* Oxford *Dictionary of English Etymology* (Oxford: Oxford University Press, 1996).
2. Margaret M. Street, *Watch—Fires on the Mountains: The Life and Writing of Ethel Johns* (Toronto: University of Toronto Press, 1975). Street won the 1973 W. S. Baird gold medal award for outstanding work in the history of health sciences for this biography.
3. Patricia D'Antonio, "Revisiting and Rethinking the Rewriting of Nursing History," *Bulletin of the History of Medicine* 73 (1999): 268–90; Christopher Maggs, "A History of Nursing: A History of Caring?" *Journal of Advanced Nursing* 23, no. 3 (1996): 632; Sioban Nelson, "The Fork in the Road: Nursing History vs. the History of Nursing?" *Nursing History Review* 10 (2002): 175.
4. Maggs, "A History of Nursing," 632; Nelson, "The Fork in the Road," 178.
5. Nelson, "The Fork in the Road," 185; Janet C. Ross Kerr, "Nursing History at the Graduate Level: State of the Art," *Canadian Bulletin of Medical History* 11, no. 1 (1994): 230.
6. Thomas H. B. Symons, quoted in Ross Kerr, "Nursing History," 232.
7. Helen Carpenter, *A Divine Discontent: Edith Kathleen Russell, Reforming Educator* (Toronto: Faculty of Nursing, University of Toronto, 1982); Natalie N. Riegler, *Jean I. Gunn: Nursing Leader* (Toronto: Queens University Press, 1997);

Judith Young, "A Divine Mission: Elizabeth McMaster and the Hospital for Sick Children, Toronto, 1875–1892," *Canadian Bulletin of Medical History* 11, no. 1 (1994): 71–90; Janet Beaton and Marion McKay, "Caroline Wellwood: Profile of a Leader," *Canadian Journal of Nursing Leadership* 12, no. 4 (1999): 30–33.

8. Ged Martin, "Foreword: Biography and History," in *Boswell's Children: The Art of the Biographer,* ed. R. B. Fleming (Toronto: Dundurn Press, 1992) ix–xv; Ross Kerr, "Nursing History," 230–33.
9. Ross Kerr, "Nursing History," 230–33.
10. "New Dissertations," *Nursing History Review* 11 (2003): 215–25.
11. Nelson, "The Fork in the Road," 178.
12. M. Louise Fitzpatrick, "Historical Research: The Method," in *Nursing Research: A Qualitative Perspective,* ed. Patricia Munhall and Carolyn Oiler Boyd, 2nd ed., (New York: National League for Nursing Press, 1993): 365; Natalie N. Riegler, "Some Issues to Be Considered in the Writing of Biography," *Canadian Bulletin of Medical History* 11 (1994): 219–20.
13. Nelson, "The Fork in the Road," 178 (emphasis added).
14. Kathleen Cruikshank, "Education History and the Art of Biography," *American Journal of Education* 107, no. 3 (1999): 231.
15. Nelson, "The Fork in the Road," 182–185.
16. Fitzpatrick, "Historical Research," 362.
17. Jacquelyn Dowd Hall, "Second Thoughts: On Writing Feminist Biography," *Feminist Studies* 13, no. 1 (1987): 23; Alice Wexler, "Emma Goldman and the Anxiety of Biography," in *The Challenge of Feminist Biography: Writing the Lives of Modern American Women,* ed. Sara Alpern, Joyce Antler, Elisabeth Israels Perry, and Ingrid Winther Scobie (Urbana: University of Illinois Press, 1992), 48.
18. Martin, "Foreword," xi.
19. Cruikshank, "Education History," 231–32.
20. Fitzpatrick, "Historical Research," 366.
21. Sir Edward Cook, noted in Riegler, "Some Issues to Be Considered," 221.
22. Cruikshank, "Education History," 238.
23. See Darlene Clark Hine, "The Ethel Johns Report: Black Women in the Nursing Profession, 1925," *Journal of Negro History* 67, no. 3 (1987): 212–28; Sonya Grypma, "Profile of a Leader: Ethel John's 'Buried' Commitment to Racial Equality, 1925," *Canadian Journal of Nursing Leadership* 16, no. 4 (1987): 39–47.
24. Elspeth Cameron, "Truth in Biography," in *Boswell's Children,* ed. R. B. Fleming, 27-32.
25. Jean Ewen, *China Nurse, 1932–1939: A Young Canadian Witnesses History* (Toronto: McClelland and Stewart, 1981).
26. Sydney Gordon and Ted Allan, *The Scalpel, the Sword: The Story of Doctor Norman Bethune,* 3rd ed. (New York: Monthly Review Press, 1973).
27. Ewen, *China Nurse,* 80; personal communication with David J. Turim, *Chicago Tribune* librarian, June 5, 2002. At my request, Turim checked the *Tribune* archives and found only two articles about Bethune—from his work in Spain (1937) and about a foreign trade exhibit (1972). He also thoroughly scanned the *Tribune* microfiche for March 12 and 13, 1938, and found that there is no such article. (It is possible that the article Ewen referred to was in a different American newspaper available in China in 1938, such as *The New York Times.*)
28. Roderick Stewart, *The Mind of Norman Bethune* (Toronto: McGraw-Hill Ryerson, 1990), 98–99. In a 1938 letter, Bethune complained that he had lost track of Ewen. Stewart writes that many years later Ewen explained that a telegram from Bethune warning her of rugged conditions kept her from returning to Sian. This differs from Ewen's explanation in *China Nurse.*

29. Fitzpatrick, "Historical Research," 367.
30. Margaret Negodaeff-Tomsik, *Honour Due: The Story of Dr. Leonora Howard King* (Ottawa: Canadian Medical Association, 1999).
31.Francess Halpenny, "Expectations of Biography," in *Boswell's Children*, ed. R. B. Fleming. 11.
32. Negodaeff-Tomsik, *Honour Due*, 86–87.
33. Alvyn Austin, *Saving China: Canadian Missionaries in the Middle Kingdom, 1888–1959* (Toronto: University of Toronto Press, 1986), 168; Grant Maxwell, "Partners in Mission: The Grey Sisters," in *Assignment in Chekiang: Seventy-One Canadians in China, 1902–1954* (Scarborough: Scarboro Foreign Mission Society, 1984), 137–138.
34. Peter Stursberg, *The Golden Hope: Christians in China* (Toronto: United Church Publishing, 1987), 60.
35. Peter Kong-ming New and Yuet-wah Cheung, "Early Years of Medical Missionary Work in the Canadian Presbyterian Mission in North Honan, China, 1887–1900," *Asian Profile* 12, no. 5 (1984): 409–423. In 1890, the Rev. James Frazer Smith, M.D., reported seeing 1,390 patients and performing 105 operations, including 10 cataracts, in a twenty-one-day period. Jonathan Goforth and Rosalyn Goforth, *Miracle Lives of China* (Grand Rapids, MI: Zondervan, 1931), vii. Goforth notes that he dictated several chapters of this book to Canadian missionary nurse Magareth Gay while "lying blindfolded after a serious eye operation."
36. Austin, *Saving China*, 168.
37. Malcolm Scott, *The China Years of Bob McClure* (Toronto: Canec, 1977).
38. Riegler, "Some Issues to be Considered," 222.
39. Elisabeth Israels Perry, "Critical Journey: From Belle Moskowitz to Women's History," in *The Challenge of Feminist Biography*, ed. S. Alpern, et al. 87.
40. Leon Edel, in Cruikshank, "Education History," 234.
41. Marc Bloch, *The Historian's Craft: Reflections on the Nature and Uses of History and the Techniques and Methods of Those Who Write It*, 5th ed., trans. Peter Putnam, 48 (Toronto: McClelland and Stewart, 1979).
42. Ibid., 50.
43. Ibid., 61–62.
44. Fitzpatrick, "Historical Research," 368.
45. Wexler, "Emma Goldman," 35–36.
46. Dee Garrison, "Two Roads Taken: Writing the Biography of Mary Heaton Vorse," in *The Challenge of Feminist Biography: Writing the Lives of Modern American Women*, ed. S. Alpern, et al., 68.
47. David A. Nock, "Biographical Truth," in *Boswell's Children*, ed. R. B. Fleming, 36.
48. Nelson, "The Fork in the Road," 180.
49. Fitzpatrick, "Historical Research," 363.
50. Leon Edel, in Cruikshank, "Education History," 233.
51. Halpenny, "Expectations of Biography," 6.
52. Cruikshank, "Education History," 233.
53. Halpenny, "Expectations of Biography," 11.
54. Gordon and Allan, *The Scalpel, the Sword*, 65, 145, 182.
55. Scott, McClure. Among other positions, McClure was a field director for the International Red Cross and worked with a Quaker-sponsored Friends Ambulance Unit on the Burma Road. According to Stursberg in *The Golden Hope*, McClure was asked by the International Red Cross to look for Bethune because he had disappeared in search of the Communist Eighth Route Army. McClure picked up his trail and led Bethune back to Tunkwan.

56. Gordon and Allan, *The Scalpel, the Sword,* 191–192.
57. Ken Mitchell, "Living the Biography, or, the Importance of Being Norman," in *Boswell's Children,* ed. R. B. Fleming, 38–44.
58. R. B. Fleming, "The Two Solitudes of History and Biography," in *Boswell's Children,* ed. R. B. Fleming, 259–66.
59. Cameron, "Truth in Biography," 30.
60. Mitchell, "The Importance of Being Norman," 40.
61. Garrison, "Two Roads Taken," 71.
62. Kathryn Kish Sklar, "Coming to Terms with Florence Kelly: The Tale of a Reluctant Biographer," in *The Challenge of Feminist Biography,*
63. Wexler, "Emma Goldman," 48.
64. Riegler, "Some Issues to Be Considered," 24.
65. Sklar, "Reluctant Biographer," 31–33.
66. Hall, "Second Thoughts," 27.
67. Cameron, "Truth in Biography," 29.
68. Janie M. Brown and Patricia D'Antonio, quoted in Ross Kerr, "Nursing History," 232.
69. Brown and D'Antonio; D'Antonio "Revisiting and Rethinking," 272.
70. D'Antonio, "Revisiting and Rethinking," 271.
71. Susan Ware, "Unlocking the Porter-Dewson Partnership: A Challenge for the Feminist Biographer," in *The Challenge of Feminist Biography,* ed. S.Alpern, et al. 51–64 (Urbana: University of Illinois Press, 1992); Hall, "Second Thoughts," 34.
72. Ware, "Feminist Biographer," 61; Hall, "Second Thoughts," 34.
73. D'Antonio, "Revisiting and Rethinking," 279.
74. Cruikshank, "Education History," 237.
75. Nelson, "The Fork in the Road," 181.
76. Ibid., 181–182.
77. Ibid., 182.
78. Cruikshank, "Education History," 231.
79. Halpenny, "Expectations of Biography," 11.
80. Leon Edel, in Cruikshank, "Education History," 235.
81. Halpenny, "Expectations of Biography," 14.
82. Cruikshank, "Education History," 234.
83. Riegler, "Some Issues to Be Considered," 222; Cruikshank, "Education History," 234; Garrison, "Two Roads Taken," 66–68.
84. Cruikshank, "Education History," 235.
85. Riegler, "Some Issues to Be Considered," 223.
86. Joan Lynaugh, "The Importance of Writing History as Narrative—Bringing Nurses and Nursing Events Alive," *Nursing History Review* 8 (2000): 1.
87. Garrison, "Two Roads Taken," 66–68.

CHAPTER SIX

Oral History Research

Geertje Boschma, Margaret Scaia, Nerrisa Bonifacio, and Erica Roberts

"Oral history is a history built around people," Paul Thompson (2000a, p. 23) noted. Tape recording conversations with people, while capturing their experiences of social developments and cultural and life events in which they took part, provides an opportunity to understand changes and occurrences from the perspective of those who experienced them. Collecting people's personal stories by tape or video recorder gained momentum as a historical research approach in the 1970s when historians, coming from a critical social stand, began to explore the voices and stories of ordinary people often overlooked in traditional historiography (Perks & Thomson, 2006; Thompson, 2000a). Oral history developed in close interdisciplinary relation with other fields in the humanities and social sciences, evolving in the interrelated approaches of oral history, life stories or life history, biography, and narrative analysis (Berger & Quinney, 2005; Bredberg, 1999; Burke, 2001; Grele, 2006; Yow, 2005).

Oral history as a historical methodology allows the narrator the freedom to express ideas and thoughts in a way that may not otherwise be preserved in a written form and about subjects that have not traditionally been topics of historical investigation (Reinharz, 1992). This freedom has its constraints, however, because the interviewer and the narrator participate in a structured but interactive process either in a single conversation, or in a series of conversations (Anderson & Jack, 2006; Biederman, 2001; Borland, 2006; Rafael, 1997; Yow, 2005). In this dynamic process of coconstructing, the narrator and interviewer engage in the creation of historical evidence, but not necessarily on an equal basis, and the relationship between interviewer and interviewee does affect the construction of the interpretation (Perks & Thomson, 2006; Sangster, 1998).

In addition to the story being recalled by the narrator, the interaction between the narrator and the researcher impacts the way the story is told, constructed, and even the themes that emerge (Borland, 2006). The oral history interview then is analyzed for meaning with attention to factors such as the standpoint of the interviewer, language structure, effects of time on past and present meaning, chronological structuring of the narrative, and social and historical context. The interviewer is an active participant in creating evidence and meaning in the research process and brings with her to the interview and its interpretation her own questions, biases, and assumptions as well as the influences of race, class, culture, education, and professional status. Listening, reading, writing, journaling, and reflecting are all part of the research design.

As the narrator recalls past events, the narration of the events and even the meaning that these events have for the narrator is affected and changed by the present telling of the story, including the environment in which the story is told, important events occurring presently for the narrator, and the nature of the relationship between the narrator and the researcher. The researcher must, in the analysis of the narrative, be sensitive to the ways in which these factors impact the narrative, and must include an analysis of these factors in the interpretation of the interview (Borland, 2006; Yow, 2005). Oral history is not merely a means of corroborating written records, but it is a source of historical testimony in its own right.

In this chapter, the authors discuss key aspects of oral history research, including issues of analysis and interpretation. They illustrate their points by using examples of their own oral history research. First, they will give a brief review of oral history approaches and discuss some unique methodological features, including sampling, consent, relying on memory, and the therapeutic potential of oral history. Then they focus on matters of analysis and interpretation of taped conversations based on examples of their own research. Boschma has been involved in two oral history projects. One oral history project involved psychiatric mental health nurses who worked in psychiatric hospitals in the Canadian province of Alberta between 1930 and 1975 (Boschma, Yonge, & Mychajlunow, 2003, 2005), and another ongoing oral history project, also in Alberta, involves family members who experienced mental illness in their family. The latter is part of a larger study on changes in mental health care in that province. Scaia (2003) completed a study that included interviews with 12 women between the ages of 18 to 80 about their experience of becoming a mother in their adolescent years between 1939 and 2001. Changes in the social and historical construction of motherhood, sexuality, and women's roles in society guided the analysis of these interviews. Bonifacio and Roberts are currently using oral history in their examination of two understudied areas of nursing's past: the history of the specialty areas of post-anesthetic care and gerontological nursing. The authors are all engaged in the intertwined tasks of posing historical questions, selecting participants, taping conversations, analyzing and interpreting the evidence, and producing a narrative, all with the purpose of contributing to the wider area of nursing and oral history scholarship.

ORAL HISTORY: MOVEMENT, METHOD, AND FRAMEWORK

Oral history then, is both a framework or analytic model and a methodology. In a comprehensive review of the field, Grele (2006) emphasizes how oral history arose as a movement with various purposes and different perspectives on the nature of the evidence it provides. Some saw oral history as a source of objective information, filling the gaps left by existing documentation, and oriented themselves to oral history as an archival practice, generating a wide range of oral history collections. Others took an activist stand, pursuing oral history as part of a new social history. From this perspective oral history serves the purpose of creating history of ordinary people's lives, not so much to complement the written record, but rather to counter the hegemonic record, the history of those in power, and to radicalize the practice of history "from the bottom up," clearly revealing its socialist origins (Grele, 2006). Kerr's (2003) collaborative analysis of homelessness "from the bottom up," empowering homeless people to speak and speak up for themselves in a collaborative effort, reflects this activist stand and social critique.

From the latter perspective, oral history can be considered a form of microhistory, or "history from below," foregrounding history from a micro rather than a macro perspective: the experience of ordinary people in their ordinary day-to-day lives (Burke, 2001; Sharpe, 2001). Oral history, Burke notes, seeks to oppose the presentation of history as grand narrative, which often represents the perspective of the most powerful, the most influential and socially dominant or ruling groups to the exclusion of the stories of the less powerful, the ordinary people, or the marginalized ones. Moreover, oral history can provide evidence of people's work and life experience of which little other written evidence exists (Biedermann, 2001).

Both these approaches to oral history share in common their relatively uncomplicated approach to the nature of telling stories, most often approaching oral history as a form of historical documentation (Grele, 2006). The increasing awareness among oral history scholars that oral history sources are narrative accounts rather than mere documentary sources marked the so-called narrative turn in oral history (Chamberlain, 2006; Grele, 2006). In storytelling, people order and reorder their past, which is mediated through life experience, memory, language, interaction, beliefs, and the broader context of life. In the interactive process of story "construction," narrator and interviewer make meaning and produce a text. Relying heavily on analytic frameworks from cultural and literary studies, oral history, in the 1980s, grew into a more socially critical and complex analytic practice (Tonkin, 1992).

Both new and seasoned nursing history scholars can now rely on an extensive oral history literature that reflects this complexity and provides guidance for the design, ethics, and interpretation of oral history. Ritchie (2003) and Yow (2005) offer a detailed discussion of oral history methodology, including ethical, legal, and design implications for individual, family, and community oral history projects. Clearly reflecting the critical social tradition of oral history, Perks and Thomson (2006) emphasize the empowering and transforming potential of oral history interviewing, giving a thorough discussion of critical developments in the field. Included in this work are directions for interviewing, interpretation, and collecting oral history, as well as discussion of its powerful digital, artistic, and performance potential. Moreover, in their recent handbook on oral history, Charlton, Myers, and Sharpless (2006) present an in-depth and critical review of the foundations, methodology, theory, and applications of oral history, including art and moving images. Several journals focus exclusively on the publication of oral history scholarship. The *Oral History Review,* the official publication of the American Oral History Association; *Oral History,* a journal based in the United Kingdom; and *Oral History Forum,* an online journal of the Canadian Oral History Association provide ongoing critical assessment of the scholarship in the field.

Bornat, Perks, Thompson, and Walmsley (2000) emphasize the value of oral history in the analysis and documentations of the "astonishing transformation of both the delivery and nature of health care and of welfare philosophies and organization in Britain and world-wide" (p. 1). Health and welfare not only play a critical role in politics and policy, but are an essential part of daily life and culture. Oral history, they argue, can help create a "more complex and rounded picture" of past health care practice, provide a perspective on private areas of life by including family and patient views and experiences, and can document the "recipient" side of health and welfare (pp. 3–4).

In collecting evidence about nurses' work and contributions to health care, oral history has been widely used in nursing history (Boschma et al., 2005; Fairman, 2002; Flynn, 2003; Rafael, 1997; Toman, 2001, 2003;

Shkimba & Flynn, 2005). Oral history is a crucial methodology in capturing nursing's past, because often nurses left behind little documentation of their work. Its potential for exploring changes in nursing and health care practice from a client point of view, however, is only in a very beginning stage. Conversations with clients and families enrich our historical understanding of health care practice in important ways and provide an area for much expansion (Boschma, in press; Cooke, 2004; Rolph, Atkinson, Mind, & Welshman, 2005; Scaia, 2003). Be it in listening to nurses or clients, oral life history accounts assist us in gaining an intimate understanding of practice dilemmas from the perspective of people who experienced them. Any oral history account, however, needs careful analysis, making use of oral history as a framework as much as a method.

Not surprisingly, in "nursing oral history," the framework or analytic model of feminist oral history has proven to be useful, because it foregrounds gender as an analytic category as well as the intersection of the categories of gender, race, and class. Because of the established perception of nursing as a field of women's work, feminist oral history provides a rich framework to understand and analyze nursing oral history. However, understanding the stories of nurses and clients can be approached from a variety of analytic models. Reflective of the complexity of oral history, most scholars draw from more than one framework, and we are no exception. Narrative and life history are also useful analytic models, and often these approaches overlap (Chamberlain, 2006; Cole & Knowles, 2001; Gluck & Patai, 1991).

As an example, feminist oral history is an approach that has distinct features, but also draws from other analytic models. Shifting the focus to women's voices and their life experiences, it evolved as a critical field of scholarship that opened up new perspectives on women's work (Gluck & Patai, 1991; Sangster, 1998). Researchers use feminist oral history for a variety of purposes. These include social advocacy for people who otherwise would not be heard in the public forum, thus recording the history of people whose stories are not usually written down. The narrator's experience is sought in all its complexity, ambiguity, and possible inconsistencies. Reinharz (1992) noted how "feminist oral histories cover extensive portions or profound experiences in an individual's life, they assist in a fundamental sociological task—illuminating the connections between biography, history, and social structure" (p. 131). Like oral history generally, feminist oral history is interdisciplinary in nature, drawing on approaches from history, psychology, sociology, and cultural studies, connecting the interrelated fields of life stories, oral history, and narrative interpretation (Anderson & Jack, 2006; Chamberlain, 2006; Gluck, 2006; Gluck & Patai, 1991; Reinharz, 1992).

Unique Features

Memory and Subjectivity

The reliance on memory in oral history has generated much controversy in the historical literature. Much debate about oral history has centered on the constructed nature of oral history evidence, questioning whether the alleged subjective historical evidence drawn from memory can be trusted (Grele, 2006; Toman, 2001). Oral historians have persuasively argued, however, that oral and written sources are equally credible (Grele, 2006; Lumis, 2006; Portelli, 2006b; Thompson, 2000a). Portelli points out that the credibility of oral history stems from its emphasis on how events are experienced rather than on providing factual accounts. The difference between oral and written sources is gradual and fluid as oral sources are turned into written ones, whereas written sources were once stories, Prins (2001) points out. No record, whether oral, written, or pictorial, speaks for itself, and always requires careful interpretation (Jordanova, 2006).

Memory "functions as an incessant work of interpretation and reinterpretation, and of organization of meaning" (Portelli, 2006a, p. 34). Memories are never a literal account of what happened, but are always a reconstruction of events and experiences. They change over time and through the process of recollection, selection, and connection with other memories (Portelli, 2006a; Sugiman, 2006). Therefore, recalling events regardless of whether they are written or oral is already an interpretation. The point of oral history is not about "lie versus truth" or whether we can get the story straight in an objective, positivistic sense, but rather how events and experiences are remembered. Amongst oral historians, memory itself has become understood as an "object of historical inquiry," moving away from a view of oral history as a source, or "set of documents that happened in people's head" (Sugiman, 2006, p. 71).

In this regard, the concept of time is also important in making sense of interview data. Sandelowski (1999) proposed a number of meta-frameworks for viewing how people reflect on events that occurred at recent and at distant points in their lives. She noted that listening to the ways that people tell their story and accounting for the ways they address change over time, "contributes to the... discovery of patterns and regularities in lives lived in time, place, and in relationships" (p. 84). It is the connection between personal and collective or public history that becomes the focus of historical inquiry. The ways in which meaning changes over time is revealed not only in the text of the story, but also in the way the story is organized chronologically, and the temporal emphasis that is placed on particular events. Memories must be subjected to the same observant historical analysis as any other primary source. Moreover, the selection of participants and sampling methods requires careful attention.

Selection and Sampling

The method of selecting participants for most oral history research projects is purposeful sampling. According to Sandelowski (1995), participation in purposeful sampling is "case-oriented" rather than "variable" oriented. That is, it is the representativeness of the experience under study that is sought, not the generalizability of the data. Purposeful sampling includes individuals on the basis of personal knowledge of the event or phenomenon, as well as the ability and willingness to communicate this experience to others (Sandalowski, 1995). The criterion for sample selection reflects the intent of the research, which for Scaia (2003), for example, was to discover and understand the social construction of women's experience of adolescent motherhood between years 1939–2001. Purposeful sampling was used to obtain a rich and varied representation of women's experience of the phenomenon over the time frame indicated. Networking and building relationships is an important aspect in purposeful sampling. Like Scaia, Boschma, Bonifacio, and Roberts build upon their relationships and networks within the respective fields of mental health, post-anesthetic, and gerontological nursing, to find the interviewees whose experience and stories can contribute to their projects. Both organized and collegial connections are important resources in finding interviewees.

Consent

Because of interviewees' participation in oral history research, ethical guidelines and regulations governing research involving human subjects have to be followed, and informed consent must be obtained prior to the start of the interview process. Researchers affiliated with colleges, universities, and health agencies must submit ethical protocols for oral history interviewing to their institutional review or ethics board (Shopes, 2006; Yow, 2005). However, this process has raised considerable debate within the oral history community. A unique aspect of oral history research is that often participants are selected because of their identity and experience, and consequently, oral history interviews are usually not anonymous and the information that the interviewee shares might not be confidential (Boschma et al., 2003; Yow, 2005).

In the late 1990s, the Oral History Association (OHA) and American History Association (AHA) developed a policy statement, arguing that "most oral history interviewing projects are not subject to...regulations for the protection of human subjects...and can be excluded from institutional review board...oversight because they do not involve research as defined by regulations of the Department of Health and Human Services (HHS)" based on the argument that the purpose of oral history is most often to illuminate the particularity of an experience rather than to contribute to generalizable knowledge, which allegedly is the underlying principle of biomedical and biobehavioral research (OHA, 2007; Shopes, 2006, p. 149). Although, in 2003, the HHS Office of Human Research Protections concurred with this policy, Shopes also points out how this policy has not become a widely accepted practice, and guidelines from local review boards may vary. Therefore, it is imperative that researchers consult with their local institutional ethics board and develop a protocol that not only meets the locally established ethical guidelines, but also fits the purposes of the oral history project. Depending on the nature of the project, protecting the identity of interviewees can be important. In Boschma's current project, for example, some family members dealing with mental illness in their family purposefully choose to not have their identity revealed. Nevertheless, their stories provide a valuable contribution to the history of the experience of living with mental illness from a family point of view and generate important insights in the historical transformation of this very process. Using pseudonyms and excluding identifiable information from the accounts can be a valid and sometimes necessary oral history research strategy.

It is important to clarify to both the reviewers of the ethical protocol and to the interviewees that consent in oral history has two aspects. First, the interviewee must be fully informed about the purpose and procedures of the oral history interview in order to provide consent to participation in the interview. Second, because most often the purpose of an oral history interview is to preserve the interview for future research and permanently store the tapes and transcripts in an existing archive or permanent oral history collection, participants must be informed about how the information is used, and they must consent to preservation and release of the interview into a permanent repository. Whether this is dealt with in a one- or a two-step process is largely a judgment call of the researchers and needs to be clearly outlined in the research protocol, and hence, in the consent forms and letters of information shared with the interviewee (Boschma et al., 2003). Shopes (2006) emphasizes how appropriate legal release and transfer of copyright is essential in making the interview accessible for future use. As part of the consent process, the range of options for handling interview recordings and transcripts must be explained to the interviewee for the purposes of the research project and for future preservation.

Therapeutic and Transformative Potential

Church and Johnson (1995) stated that the process of oral history includes therapeutic dimensions. In their oral history project with psychiatric mental health nurses, Boschma et al. (2003) observed how the reminiscing that occurred in the interviews sometimes provoked strong emotions or brought up unresolved issues. "Some interviewees looked back on experiences with mixed feelings because what seemed common and accepted approaches at the time, were now viewed in a negative light. Others grieved for the work life they had enjoyed and that had been a central part of their lives," they noted (p. 131). Because of the unique nature of personal accounts, which are closely related to art and imagination, the process of telling stories lends itself to therapeutic purposes, and this empowering effect can thus have a therapeutic application.

Reminiscence and life history approaches have obtained an established place in health and social work with older people, encouraging them to recall and reflect on experiences and events in their past (Bornat, 1999). Bornat (2006) has outlined the similarities and differences in reminiscence and oral history, especially in relation to life review, memory, and dealing with traumatic experiences. Bornat suggests that reminiscence has the potential to raise self-worth through the legitimizing effect of telling personal stories.

This therapeutic dimension can also be employed as a resource in bringing the oral history interview to a closure. This process can include simple, but important gestures such as asking how the interviewee has experienced the interview and thanking the interviewee for their contribution. We have found that taking a brief moment to debrief toward the end of the interview is a valuable part of the interview process (Boschma et al., 2003).

ORAL HISTORY: PURPOSE AND INTERPRETATION

As outlined previously, presenting oral testimony can have very different purposes (Grele, 2006; Thompson, 2000a). In our work, we draw on all three traditions of oral history, recapped by Grele. Our projects include the goal of preserving nurses' oral testimony about their work experiences and participation in important changes in health care. Second, the emancipatory goal of presenting voices and perspectives of those who intimately experienced life events of health and illness, whether that is from the perspective of health care recipients or nurses, is reflected in our work. Third, all of our projects are reflective of narrative analysis and interpretation, informed by recent oral history scholarship.

Preservation of nurses' stories can be an objective in and of itself, especially if nurses have work experiences in an area of health care that is rapidly changing. Moreover, certain areas of nursing work are more emphasized than others when the historical role of nursing in health care is highlighted. Nurses' work in mental health care, for example, has long been an understudied area in nursing history (Boschma, 2003). This observation formed in part the background for an oral history project that Boschma et al. (2003, 2005) conducted with psychiatric mental health nurses in Alberta, Canada. It had the specific purpose to highlight important transformations in psychiatric mental health care from the vantage point of nurses. The project was designed to preserve nursing history by recording the personal narratives of nurses who cared for mentally ill patients in either institutional settings or community services between 1940 and 1993. The project generated a unique collection of primary source materials, allowing for a critical examination of nurses' past contributions to mental health care and of the interface between their work and the broader social and political context of mental health care.

In preserving life stories, whether individually or as a collection of stories, the emphasis is on the story as told by the narrators (Thompson, 2000a). Upon the completion of the interviews, however, once the researcher begins to analyze and interpret the stories, the process of coconstruction halts, and the story becomes that of the historian. "Although the telling of the story can be framed as co-creating, suggesting a shared initiative, or even sharing of power, once the 'listener' turns into an 'interpreter', the 'voice' becomes that of the professional historian," Sangster (1998, pp. 92–93) points out. From an analysis of selected interviews with psychiatric mental health nurses for example, Boschma et al. (2005) observed how the development of psychiatric nurses' professional identity intersected with gender in the construction of psychiatric nursing practice. Although the nurses did not frame their experience in terms of gender, close analysis of their stories about their work and the changes in care in which they took part led the researchers to argue that the accounts did reveal how gender had structured the nurses' experience, linking the individual story to larger social changes. Narrative interpretation seeks to understand how the subjective, individual experiences of ordinary people are both shaped by and exemplars of larger social processes, but the interpretation offered is that of the researcher.

Historical interpretation, Thompson (2000a) notes, has a stronger emphasis on analysis, whether that is a narrative analysis or a reconstructive cross-analysis. In the latter, the purpose is to "construct an argument about patterns of behaviour or events in the past" (p. 271), which may include an analysis of demographic or other numerical data. In narrative analysis, on the other hand, the interview is treated as a text and concerns itself with "language, its themes and repetitions, and its silences, [and] how the narrator experienced, remembered, and retold his or her life-story, and what light this may throw on the consciousness of the wider society" (p. 270). In the remainder of the chapter we will further illustrate how narrative interpretation of personal accounts, either from mothers, family members, or nurses, can foster a critical understanding of our collective consciousness and broader disciplinary discourses around important life experiences, such as adolescent motherhood and dealing with mental illness, as well as the construction of disciplinary nursing knowledge and practice.

ORAL HISTORY FROM A "RECIPIENT" POINT OF VIEW

Scaia' 2003 research around the history of adolescent motherhood was in part driven by her insight that nurses' disciplinary knowledge base would be enhanced by a fuller understanding of the constructed nature of adolescent motherhood, as revealed in oral history accounts of mother (Scaia, 2003). The experience of motherhood is both a private and public act and one in which nurses often play an important role. While motherhood was once an event that occurred almost exclusively within the context of marriage, the stories from the women Scaia interviewed revealed how changes in women's lives over the past 60 years have meant the decision to mother is now a reflection of the values and beliefs of the woman making the decision to mother rather than an expectation of the outcome of marriage. In light of these changes, it is important for nurses to understand historical transformations in the way that society evaluates motherhood and what it means to be a woman and a mother.

Beliefs and assumptions about what it means to be a nurse have also changed over the past decades. While certain nursing perspectives might once have been identified as typical of all nurses 60 years ago, today, the emphasis on the individual has meant that each nurse brings with her a unique perspective that is shaped by the particular social and historical context in which she lived. Nursing practices are thus individually situated, and nurses expect to have these perspectives respected. In working with young women who may or may not be married, be financially independent, or from a similar cultural background, it is important to examine the ways in which nurses' attitudes toward women at this vulnerable point in their life are formed and how they influence nurses' care.

Scaia (2003) focused on the perspective of clients rather than nurses in her exploration of changes in personal and social attitudes over time in relation to adolescent motherhood. In this process of interpretation, she was able to contextualize the notion and image of teenage motherhood as a historically constructed event. In one account for example, she co-constructed the experience of being an adolescent and being a mother with Ellen (pseudonym), a young woman who had her first child at the age of 16 in 2000. In this account, Ellen wondered if the image of the bad girl and the pregnant teenager will ever be erased from the social mythology of Western middle-class society. She feels that society still fears women's sexuality and, particularly, the teenage woman's sexuality. This is one reason, she believes, that adults stereotype young unmarried mothers and don't want to hear about their individual experiences of motherhood, or find out what they might learn from them about mothering. According to Wong and Checkland (1999), the image of "children having children"—implying children having sex—is disturbing to many who have lingering associations about the immorality of sex outside marriage. Ellen responded thoughtfully:

> I don't know. I have been trying to figure out what they've been talking about when they, when people talk about teenage pregnancy. Some people think it's wrong to have sex when you were a teenager in the first place, which is... I don't know if it's the unmarried thing or the teenage thing because most of the same people don't think that there is anything wrong with having sex when you're older, although there are a lot of people who do, but, they seem to think if you get pregnant and they have this... stereotype of what you must be like, and the thing is that it's hard because a lot of people have sex and they don't all get pregnant, and why are you only biased against the ones who get pregnant? They say, you know, "well, it's her fault because she was a slut or she fucks around" or whatever she did. (Interview transcript #2, Ellen, pp. 7–8)

In this statement, Ellen challenges the ways in which beliefs about women and sex are shaped by a particular social and historical context. In the past, having a child in the teenage years was not unusual, as long as the woman was married. In recounting her experience of being a mother in her teenage years in 2000, Ellen explores how social and historical changes in women's roles in society have impacted the experience of early motherhood. In revealing her thoughts and feelings about this experience, and the ways in which she feels judged and evaluated as an unmarried teenage mother, Ellen reveals the potential negative and hurtful impact of lingering attitudes by the dominant society—including nurses—about women, sexuality, and motherhood. Inclusion of these insights through the use of feminist oral history serves to raise awareness among nurses and other health professionals about assumptions we possibly make. Critical reflection upon such assumptions might enhance a more sensitive approach to young women experiencing early childbirth and motherhood.

How family members have experienced mental illness in their family, how they responded to health services, and how they helped shape health services is at the heart of Boschma's current research (Boschma, in press-*a*). As part of this project, she conducts oral history interviews with family members who experienced mental illness in their family, sometimes over multiple generations (Boschma, in press-*b*). The purpose of her study is—rephrasing Thompson (2000a)—to explore how family members "retold, remembered and experienced" their family life, of which mental illness was part (p. 270). Using oral history accounts, she aims to explore what family members' stories reveal about the broader, cultural discourse on mental illness that shapes their individual experiences. The stories are analyzed as text and testimony, but the emphasis of the interpretation is on what the language used by the participants conveys about the experience. The narrative interpretation of these oral histories throws light upon the ways family members actively participate in the construction of mental health care as they accommodate to and resist the dominant discourse on mental illness.

Rosenberg (2002) and Kleinman (1988) point out how the biomedical framing of disease as a specific entity, with a specific, identifiable cause, diagnosis, and treatment or therapy, is central to current social and cultural understanding of mental illness. The oral histories Boschma conducted with family members reveal how people relate to this dominant view of mental illness in very different ways, varying from accommodation to resistance (Boschma, in press-*b*). The way memories are shared and the language in which people express themselves in the interview gives an indication of the way a narrator relates to dominant discourses and ideologies. Pat's story of her mother, who suffered from mental illness since the time Pat was a child, illustrates how Pat framed her mother's life in a way that suggests resistance to the dominant discourse. Pat said:

> I don't know, you never know what the problem is, you know from, why are they that way? But I still often think of it and I don't think she had schizophrenia. I think it was her life. (Boschma, in press-*b*)

What Pat remembered about her mother and how she had experienced her mother during her childhood could not adequately be captured in the dominant medical discourse of mental illness. For Pat, her mother had always been a good mother who had stayed faithful to her family despite the odds of an abusive husband, severe poverty during the Depression and Second World War era, and a restless existence. Her mother's commitment to her children stood out for Pat as a story of ability, not disability. In carefully listening to Pat, to her silences as much as to what she has to say or is able to say (Passerini, 1992; Portelli, 2006b), we learn about a counter-narrative quietly but persistently maintained in the face of a dominant discourse. We actually see ways in which Pat challenges such a discourse (Thompson, 2000b).

RECONSTRUCTING NURSING PRACTICE AND KNOWLEDGE

Bonifacio and Roberts had pertinent questions about their practice that they felt could be best answered using historical methods. Bonifacio's interest in historical research stems from her practice as a post-anesthetic nurse. The post-anesthetic recovery room is a specialized and designated unit where a patient recovers from a surgical procedure and the effects of anesthesia. She wondered about the ongoing controversy surrounding family visitation in the recovery room. Nursing literature dating back to the mid-1980s challenged the practice of restricting family visitation during the immediate post-operative phase. However, despite a growing body of evidence over the past 20 years in support of family visitation in the post-anesthetic recovery room, in her day-to-day practice she noticed family visitation had remained a controversial phenomenon. How had this practice historically been constructed? Why was it still controversial today?

In exploring the evolution of family visitation policy, little archival documentation could be found. Oral histories became a crucial primary source. It is a powerful tool to unearth the meaning of past events and experiences from an individual who possesses firsthand knowledge (Biedermann, 2001). Bonifacio interviewed nine registered nurses who possessed firsthand knowledge and experience working in an adult post-anesthetic recovery room during the 1960s–1980s in the Greater Vancouver area.

A reoccurring theme that surfaced during these oral history interviews was the issue of space. This concept seemed worth exploring as one explanatory context of the restriction of family visitation in the recovery room. The literal lack of physical space in the recovery room, as well as the symbolic meaning of the recovery room as a safe space, formed the most important legitimizations for nurses to restrict family visitation. One, Nurse SF, stated:

> It's a factor of space...I would say that is the biggest thing because...there's no more than this amount of space...about four feet between the beds...And so the nurse is between the beds and...he or she is trying to do charting and has equipment there and so there just really isn't that much space. (Interview #5, p. 9)

Lack of space and lack of privacy was on the minds of the nurses when they talked about reasons why family members did not fit in easily. Nurse LM noted: "there was very little space, I mean the beds were quite close together, there was no privacy" (Interview #6, p. 18). The nurses' responses helped explain how and why the recovery room functioned in a particular manner and how nurses dealt with matters of family involvement. Their comments reflected a deeper symbolic meaning of physical space (Adams, 1996; Elliot, 2004; Kingsley, 1988). In their descriptions of a physical environment not conducive to family members, they constructed a concept of space that represented safety. To them safety meant providing safe and competent nursing care to the patient. Safety of the patient was the main priority of the nurses, as patients were admitted in the recovery room with a number of postoperative complications and, if left unattended, could result in death. Constant and frequent observation and assessment of the patient was of utmost importance. Family members did not fit in easily, literally and symbolically. Historical analysis revealed how the idea of restricted family visitation matched deep felt beliefs and practices of daily nursing routines and technologies of adult recovery room care and made sense in the context of the time of the early development of the recovery room.

In reconstructing past practices, nurse historians often face the situation that little documentation has been left behind about particular changes in health care or about the responses or accommodations to them. Roberts' oral history study of nurse educator's experiences in developing gerontological nursing reflects that dilemma. As an experienced gerontological nurse with an extensive career in nursing care for older adults, Roberts noticed that many of the nurses working in those settings, particularly newly graduated nurses, seemed to lack some of the necessary knowledge needed to care for older adults. What were the difficulties in adequately preparing new recruits in this area? Anecdotal reports from other gerontological nurses and evidence from the nursing literature (Baumbusch & Goldenberg, 2000; Earthy, 1993; Kaasalainen et al., 2006; Pringle, 1983; Rosenfeld, Bottrell, Fulmer, & Mezey, 1999) indicated similar concerns about inadequate preparation of new graduates in nursing care to older adults. Roberts wanted to know why, in spite of the current demographics and the recognition of gerontological nursing as a specialty, nursing lags behind other professions' inclusion of gerontology in their educational curricula (Mahoney, 1993). Despite a beginning history of gerontological nursing and education (Davis, 1971; Ebersole, Hess, Touhy, & Jett, 2005; Mahoney, 1993), it is not well understood why such a lag exists. Mentoring in the workplace has played a predominant role in the professional growth and development of gerontological nursing (Ebersole et al., 2005). It seemed to have been developed from a grassroots level.

In order to understand the complexities around the inclusion of gerontology in basic nursing curricula and the understanding of gerontological nursing itself, a historical approach to examining the development of gerontology and its relation to nursing education is vital. Hamilton (1993) states that "for nursing, an understanding of the profession's past can provide an analysis of its beliefs, its leaders, its institutions and its work in a way that demonstrates that nursing, as a set of ideas, is a living force of continuous existence" (p. 45). There is little in the literature describing the experiences and perceptions of educators who have been involved in developing and promoting gerontology as a legitimate and necessary field of nursing knowledge and study.

Oral history evidence enables further understanding of the barriers that prevent inclusion of gerontological nursing in undergraduate programs on an equal footing with other subspecialty areas. One nurse's account in Roberts' study illustrates the interacting forces of social values regarding aging and nursing work. This nurse had taken a 20-year break from nursing and then returned to work after a refresher course. She described the attitude taken toward returning nurses:

> You're second class because you've been out of nursing, you gave it up, you've now come back, well, you've sort of lost some of those skills although we've tried to teach you, you're up to date and that. Yes, you were second class. (Interview #1)

Her experience with finding employment clearly revealed the social values regarding older adults and their care:

> When I looked for employment after that [course], they suggested, well you've been out for awhile, you know, you'll do less harm if you go into gerontology because they're old and they're going to die anyway, they've had their lives. (Interview #1)

This nurse's story is a powerful illustration of what was unofficially or informally happening "behind the scenes." Officially, this nurse was duly registered with her licensing body and therefore was legally considered capable of practicing nursing in any health care area. Formal documents from the time would reflect this fact. However, as this example shows, oral history brings out another dimension of the situation and reveals some of the interacting cultural and social forces that shaped nursing care of older adults. A better historical understanding of those forces might assist gerontological nurses in their efforts to further develop the field.

CONCLUSION: WHY USE ORAL HISTORY?

As Thompson (2000b) noted, many existing historical records give the point of view of people in authority. In contrast, oral history contributes to a historical analysis that might challenge established and accepted accounts and provide a fuller reconstruction of the past, opening up important new areas of inquiry while adding new and vivid historiography. "Oral sources tell us not just what people did, but what they wanted to do, what they believed they were doing, and what they now think they did" (Portelli, 2006b, p. 36). They allow us a peek "behind the scenes," as Roberts pointed out. Moreover, they provide documentation of changes and practice experiences in health care of which little other documentation exists.

Using the framework of feminist oral history, Scaia's (2003) analysis of women's experience of having a baby during their teenage years unsettles taken-for-granted views and assumptions about teenage motherhood, linking individual stories to larger social and cultural changes in women's and families' lives. Such a narrative can enrich nurses' knowledge base, she argues. Bonifacio illustrates how nurses' stories about the changing practice of post-anesthetic care, if carefully interpreted, provide a context in which the tension around family visitation can be understood. Oral histories, Roberts notes, capture gerontological nurse educators' experiences and the social pressures placed upon them, reflecting larger social constraints on care of the elderly. Boschma's analysis of family members' accounts of their families' experience with mental illness reveals ambivalent responses to the dominant frameworks that structure psychiatric care, mirroring the wider complexity, if not social uneasiness of dealing with mental illness. Oral history, we argue, can contribute to a critical understanding of nursing practice and inform the frameworks we use to analyze and critique nursing and health care, enriching its historical understanding. Continuous reflection upon the theoretical underpinnings as well as the methodological implications of the approach is an intrinsic part of the endeavor.

REFERENCES

Adams, A. (1996). *Architecture in the family way.* Montreal, Quebec & Kingston, Ontario: McGill-Queen's University Press.

Anderson, K., & Jack, D. C. (2006). Learning to listen: Interview techniques and analysis. In R. Perks & A. Thomson (Eds.), *The oral history reader* (2nd ed., pp. 129–142). London: Routledge.

Baumbusch, J. L., & Goldenberg, D. (2000). The impact of an aging population on curriculum development in Canadian undergraduate nursing education. *Perspectives, 24*(2), 8–14.

Berger, R. J., & Quinney, R. (2005). The narrative turn in social inquiry. In R. J. Berger and R. Quinney (Eds.), *Storytelling sociology. Narrative as social inquiry* (pp. 1–10). Boulder, CO: Lynne Rienner Publishers.

Biedermann, N. (2001). The voices of days gone by: Advocating the use of oral history in nursing. *Nursing Inquiry, 8,* 61–62.

Borland, K. (2006). "That's not what I said": Interpretive conflict in oral narrative research. In R. Perks & A. Thomson (Eds.), *The oral history reader* (2nd ed., pp. 310–321). London: Routledge.

Bornat, J. (Ed.). (1999). *Biographical interviews: The link between research and practice.* London: Centre for Policy on Aging.

Bornat, J. (2006). Reminiscence and oral history: Parallel universes or shared endeavour? In R. Perks & A. Thomson (Eds.), *The oral history reader* (2nd ed., pp. 456–473). London: Routledge.

Bornat, J., Perks, R., Thompson, P., & Walmsley, J. (Eds.). (2000). *Oral history, health and welfare.* London: Routledge.

Boschma, G. (2003). *The rise of mental health nursing: A history of psychiatric care in Dutch asylums, 1890–1920.* Amsterdam: Amsterdam University Press.

Boschma, G. (in press-*a*). A family point of view: Negotiating asylum care in Alberta, 1905–1930. *Canadian Bulletin for the History of Medicine.*

Boschma, G. (in press-*b*). Accommodation and resistance to the dominant cultural discourse on psychiatric mental health: Oral history accounts of family members. *Nursing Inquiry.*

Boschma, G., Yonge, O., & Mychajlunow, L. (2003). Consent in oral history interviews: Unique challenges. *Qualitative Health Research, 13*(1), 129–135.

Boschma, G., Yonge, O., & Mychajlunow, L. (2005). Gender and professional identity in psychiatric nursing practice in Alberta, Canada, 1930–1975. *Nursing Inquiry, 12*(4), 243–255.

Bredberg, E. (1999). Writing disability history: Problems, perspectives and sources. *Disability and Society, 14*(2), 189–201.

Burke, P. (2001). History of events and the revival of narrative. In P. Burke (Ed.), *New perspectives on historical writing* (2nd ed., pp. 283–300). Cambridge, UK: Polity Press.

Chamberlain, M. (2006). Narrative theory. In T. L. Charlton, L. E. Myers, & R. Sharpless (Eds.), *Handbook of oral history* (pp. 384–410). Lanham, MD: AltaMira Press.

Charlton, T. L., Myers, L. E., & Sharpless, R. (Eds.). (2006). *Handbook of oral history.* Lanham, MD: AltaMira Press.

Church, O. M., & Johnson, M. L. (1995). Worth remembering: The process and products of oral history. *International History of Nursing Journal, 1*(1), 19–31.

Cole, A. L., & Knowles, J. G. (Eds.). (2001). *Lives in context: The art of life history research.* New York: AltaMira Press.

Cooke, D. (2004). *Understanding schizophrenia and relapse from persons who experience it: An oral history.* Unpublished Master's Thesis in Nursing. University of Calgary, Calgary, Canada.

Davis, B. A. (1971). Geriatric nursing through the looking glass. *Journal of the New York State Nurses Association, 2*(3), 7–12.

Earthy, A. E. (1993). A survey of gerontological curricula in Canada: Generic baccalaureate nursing programs. *Journal of Gerontological Nursing, 19*(12), 7–14.

Ebersole, P., Hess, P., Touhy, T., & Jett, K. (2005). *Gerontological nursing and healthy aging* (2nd ed.). St Louis, MO: Elsevier Mosby.

Elliot, J. (2004). Blurring the boundaries of space: Shaping nursing lives at the Red Cross outposts in Ontario, 1922–1945. *Canadian Bulletin of Medical History, 21*(2), 303–325.

Fairman, J. (2002). The roots of collaborative practice: Nurse practitioners pioneers' stories. *Nursing History Review, 10,* 159–174.

Flynn, K. (2003). Race, the state and Caribbean immigrant nurses, 1950–1962. In G. Feldberg, M. Ladd-Taylor, A. Li, & K. McPherson (Eds.), *Women, health and nation: Canada and the United States since 1945* (pp. 247–263). Montreal and Kingston: McGill-Queen's University Press.

Gluck, S. B. (2006). Women's oral history: Is it so special? In T. L. Charlton, L. E. Myers, & R. Sharpless (Eds.), *Handbook of oral history* (pp. 357–383). Lanham, MD: AltaMira Press.

Gluck, S. B., & Patai, D. (Eds.). (1991). *Women's words: The feminist practice of oral history.* New York: Routledge.

Grele, R. J. (2006). Oral history as evidence. In T. L. Charlton, L. E. Myers, & R. Sharpless (Eds.), *Handbook of oral history* (pp. 43–101). Lanham, MD: AltaMira Press.

Hamilton, D. B. (1993). The idea of history and the history of ideas. *Image: Journal of Nursing Scholarship, 25*(1), 45–48.

Jordanova, L. (2006). *History in practice* (2nd ed.). London: Hodder Arnold.

Kaasalainen, S., Baxter, P., Martin, L. S., Prentice, D., Rivers, S., D'Hondt, A., et al. (2006). Are new graduates prepared for gerontological nursing practice? Current perceptions and future directions. *Perspectives, 30*(1), 4–10.

Kerr, D. (2003). "We know what the problem is": Using oral history to develop a collaborative analysis of homelessness from the bottom up. *Oral History Review, 30*(1), 27–45.

Kingsley, K. (1988). The architecture of nursing. In A. H. Jones (Ed.), *Images of nurses: Perspectives from history, art, and literature* (pp. 63–94). Philadelphia: University of Pennsylvania.

Kleinman, A. (1988). What is a psychiatric diagnosis? In A. Kleinman (Ed.), *Rethinking psychiatry: From cultural category to personal experience* (pp. 5–17). New York: The Free Press and Macmillan.

Lumis, R. (2006). Structure and validity in oral evidence. In R. Perks & A. Thomson (Eds.), *The oral history reader* (2nd ed., pp. 255–260). London: Routledge.

Mahoney, D. F. (1993). Gerontology in the nursing curriculum: Evolution and issues. *Gerontology and Geriatrics Education, 13*(3), 85–97.

Oral History Association. (2007). *Oral history excluded from Institutional Review Board (IRB) review. Policy statement on human subjects research.* Retrieved June 18, 2007, from http://omega.dickinson.edu/organizations/oha/org_irb.html

Passerini, L. (1992). Introduction. In L. Passerini (Ed.), *International yearbook of oral history and life stories. Memory and totalitarianism* (Vol. 1, pp. 1–19). Oxford: Oxford University Press.

Perks, R., & Thomson, A. (Eds.). (2006). *The oral history reader* (2nd ed.). London: Routledge.

Portelli, A. (2006a). So much depends on a red bus, or innocent victims of the liberating gun. *Oral History, 34*(2), 29–43.

Portelli, A. (2006b). What makes oral history different. In R. Perks & A. Thomson (Eds.), *The oral history reader* (2nd ed., pp. 32–42). London: Routledge.

Pringle, D. (1983). Issues and challenges confronting gerontological nursing. In E. Gallagher, M. Jackson, & G. Zilm (Eds.), *Proceedings of the First National Conference on Gerontological Nursing, Vol. II: Special Needs, Extraordinary Challenges* (pp. 171–179). Victoria, BC, Canada: University of Victoria School of Nursing.

Prins, G. (2001). Oral history. In P. Burke (Ed.), *New perspectives on historical writing* (2nd ed., pp. 120–156). Cambridge, UK: Polity Press.

Rafael, A. R. (1997). Advocacy oral history: A research methodology for social criticism in nursing. *Advances in Nursing Science, 20*(2), 32–44.

Reinharz, S. (1992). *Feminist methods in social research.* New York: Oxford University Press.

Ritchie, D. A. (2003). *Doing oral history: A practical guide.* New York: Oxford University Press.

Rolph, S., Atkinson, D., Mind, M., & Welshman, J. (Eds.). (2005). *Witnesses to change: Families, learning difficulties and history.* Kidderminster, UK: BILD Publications.

Rosenberg, C. E. (2002). The tyranny of diagnosis: Specific entities and individual experience. *The Millbank Quarterly, 80*(2), 237–260.

Rosenfeld, P., Bottrell, M., Fulmer, T., & Mezey. M. (1999). Gerontological nursing content in baccalaureate nursing programs: Findings from a national survey. *Journal of Professional Nursing, 15*(2), 84–94.

Sandelowski, M. (1995). Focus on qualitative methods: Sample size in qualitative research. *Nursing and Health, 18,* 179–183.

Sandelowski, M. (1999). Time and qualitative research. *Research in Nursing and Health, 22,* 79–87.

Sangster, J. (1998). Telling our stories: Feminist debates and the use of oral history. In R. Perks & A. Thomson (Eds.), *The oral history reader* (1st ed., pp. 87–100). London: Routledge.

Scaia, M. (2003). Understanding the experience of adolescent motherhood, 1939–2001. Unpublished Master's thesis in nursing, University of Calgary, Calgary, Canada.

Sharpe, J. (2001). History from below. In P. Burke (Ed.), *New perspectives on historical writing* (pp. 24–41). Cambridge, UK: Polity Press.

Shkimba, M., & Flynn, K. (2005). "In England we did nursing": Caribbean and British nurses in Great Britain and Canada, 1950–1970. In B. Mortimer & S. McGann (Eds.), *New directions in the history of nursing* (pp. 141–157). London: Routledge Taylor & Francis Group.

Shopes, L. (2006). Legal and ethical issues in oral history. In T. L. Charlton, L. E. Myers, & R. Sharpless (Eds.), *Handbook of oral history* (pp. 135–169). Lanham, MD: AltaMira Press.

Sugiman, P. (2006). "These feelings that fill my heart": Japanese Canadian women's memories of internment. *Oral History, 34*(2), 69–84, especially pp. 71 and 82.

Thompson, P. (2000a). *The voice of the past: Oral history* (3rd ed.). Oxford, UK: Oxford University Press.

Thompson, P. (2000b). Introduction. In J. Bornat, R. Perks, P. Thompson, & J. Walmsley (Eds.), *Oral history, health and welfare* (pp. 1–21). London: Routledge.

Toman, C. (2001). Blood work: Canadian nursing and blood transfusion, 1942–1990. *Nursing History Review, 9,* 51–78.

Toman, C. (2003). *Officers and ladies: Canadian nursing sisters, women's work, and the Second World War.* Unpublished doctoral dissertation in history, University of Ottawa, Ottawa, Canada.

Tonkin, E. (1992). *Narrating our pasts: The social construction of oral history.* Cambridge, UK: Cambridge University Press.

Wong, J., & Checkland, D. (Eds.). (1999). *Teen pregnancy and parenting.* Toronto: University of Toronto Press.

Yow, V. R. (2005). *Recording oral history: A guide for the humanities and social sciences.* Walnut Creek: AltaMira Press.

CHAPTER SEVEN

Reflections on Researcher Subjectivity and Identity in Nursing History

Geertje Boschma, Sonya J. Grypma, and Florence Melchior

"Oral historians are well aware that subjectivity—both our subject's and our own—shapes the content and interpretation of our work," Chandler (2005, p. 48) recently observed. Whereas Chandler focused in particular on the influence of age and generational differences between interviewer and interviewee in oral history, we believe her argument has wider implications. How are we, as subjects, involved in our historical interpretation? The specific question we pose for this chapter is: how do we as nurse historians construct our stories? Nurse historians heavily rely on the broader fields of social and women's history as a context or framework for their interpretations, clearly identifying with the work and approaches of historians. Yet, we wonder how we, as nurses, are involved in our historical research? Does our positioning as nurses affect the choice of our topic? Does our nursing background inform our analyses and interpretations? As nursing history gains increasing attention in historiography, it seems timely to explore these larger methodological questions

An earlier version of this chapter was presented at the Annual Conference of the Canadian Association for the History of Nursing, St. Paul's Hospital, Vancouver, BC, June 8–10, 2006. The research for this chapter was supported in part by funding from the Canadian Social Sciences and Humanities Research Council (SSHRC standard research grant no. 410–2003–1882, and a SSHRC post-doctoral fellowship).

about the reciprocity of history and nursing (D'Antonio, 2006). In this chapter, we reflect on our subjectivity and identity as nurses in our historical research, drawing on some examples from our own work.

An interpretation, whether of a written record or of evidence generated by the researcher in oral histories, is always a particular one, reflecting the subjective position of the researcher. Methodological debates in the social sciences have long emphasized the subjective nature of interpretation and the influence the researcher has on the construction of evidence in recorded interviews and participant observation. We bring many "selves" to the research. Reinharz (1997), in a reflection upon the role of the self in (social scientific) field work, proposes "that we both *bring* the self to the field and *create* the self in the field. The self we create *in the field* is a product of the norms of the social setting and the ways in which the 'research subjects' interact with the selves the researcher brings *to the field*" (p. 3). Over the last few decades, the subjectivity of historical interpretation and positioning of the researcher has become a pivotal argument (Burke, 2001). The idea that a historian provides a neutral, objective analysis that reveals "the truth" about past events has grown increasingly controversial (Wall, 2006). The selection of topics has also changed. According to Burke, human experiences and activities of a more subjective nature, which were once overlooked by historians, are now thought of as historically situated and thus fair subjects for historical analysis. Topics such as death, madness, the body, femininity, speaking, and even silence can be subjected to historical analysis, Burke notes, adding, "the philosophical foundation of the new history is the idea that reality is socially or culturally constructed" (p. 3). Each human experience is different, constructed in a particular time, place, and context.

Post-structural critics have furthered the analysis of the subjective point of view in historiography. For example, the main goal of Foucault's project was to explain the subjection of human beings: "[Foucault's] objective [...] has been to create a history of the different modes [of objectivation] by which, in our culture, human beings are made subjects" (Dreyfus & Rabinow, 1982, p. 208). A "woman" or a "nurse" is not a self-evident identity, but rather a subjected being—made, constructed, or acculturated in a particular category. Presenting ourselves as certain beings implies admitting to be caught up in a certain historical construction, a category that is situated in time and place. Riley (1988), in her well-known work on feminism and the category of "women" in history, provided a salient reflection on exactly that dilemma: Am I That Name? Language, hegemonic (world) views, culture, and history shape us and the categories in which we seek to express ourselves. Some categories we "belong" to are not perceived as matters of choice—for example, we are born as male or female. Others are perceived as choice—such as choosing to become a nurse or a historian. Even so, these choices can be perceived as a reproduction of many social and cultural influences. In enacting to be a nurse or historian we negotiate each category by constructing, reproducing, and reconstructing its meaning as well as our understanding of the skill and practice connected to each. Being both historian and nurse necessarily means these categories intersect.

PHILOSOPHICAL QUESTIONS

Subjectivity, according to one philosophical dictionary, pertains "to the subject and his or her particular perspective, feelings, beliefs, and desires" (Sol, 1995, p. 857). Reflecting on subjectivity, or what it means to be a particular subject in our work, raises several different philosophical questions. We will emphasize questions from three philosophical perspectives: post-structuralist, phenomenological, and epistemological (Sol, 1995).

Post-Structuralist

From a post-structural point of view, we must ask the question, what does it mean to be categorized? To be subjected to a certain category? What does it mean that, as researchers, we are subjected to a general idea of *researcher*? Or, using Foucault's perspective to articulate the point: what modes of objectivation and disciplinary techniques construct us into the researchers we are? For example, if "cultural coding" of masculinity and femininity shaped nurses' professional identity in a particular way—linking it to particular masculine and feminine values—does such coding not also affect nurses who do historical research? (Davis, 1995, pp. 26–27). "Cultural coding" happens in a relational context of power, negotiation, accommodation, and resistance. The "hegemonic effect" of any culturally dominant discourse, then, is a culturally produced effect, shaped, sustained, formed, and (re)produced within a complex network of human interaction (Davis, 1995; Mol, 2006).

We might be able to resist being framed or positioned in a certain category, but we cannot escape our situatedness, our positioning within an interactional network of power relations or effects. Exploring subjectivity then, is a crucial strategy to understand the complexity of many different and opposing voices with which we speak. "Nurse" is a category with a history that precedes us. Thus, becoming a nurse means becoming acculturated in an already existing field. Our interpretations, no matter how genuine and trustworthy, come with a catch. We can articulate neither our knowledge nor our experiences independently from the hegemonic narratives we have been acculturated into—the very narratives we may seek to avoid.

Phenomenological

From a phenomenological point of view, we can ask what it is like to be a certain being (e.g., woman, nurse, and historian [Sol, 1995]). What selves, emotions, and experiences do we bring to our interpretations? Do our experiences as nurses carry over into our historical interpretations? If so, how? Our experiences shape us as readers, listeners, and interpreters in particular ways, influencing the questions we ask and the subjects we choose (Chandler, 2005). Do interviewees talk differently to an interviewer who is a nurse? Who we are as subjects may allow us to see certain things while blinding us to others.

Epistemological

Finally, the notion of subjectivity in historiography raises epistemological questions. How are we positioned as *knowers* in our interpretation? We face an epistemological dilemma in being a subject in our (scientific) work. The question of how we come to certain, objective knowledge has preoccupied generations of philosophers and scholars since the time of Descartes' *Cogito ergo sum* (Sol, 1995). We speak from an "I" position while actively constructing scientific knowledge. Such knowledge is neither neutral nor objective. Scientific or historical accounts claiming to represent a perspective pertaining to all human beings, in reality often pertained to particular human beings—for example, white males. This particular blindness excluded women and people of color from the historic record, concealing from view the gendered and racialized construction of whiteness (Harding, 2001). The deconstruction of whiteness as a racialized notion is a relatively recent historical argument, furthered amongst others by feminist scholars (Frankenberg, 1993; Roediger, 1999).

The construction of nurses as white, female, and middle class has dominated much of modern nursing's history. It is a salient example of a larger dominant, hegemonic paradigm, centered in the West. Nurses had an essential role in constructing and enacting such views—something nurse historians recently began to recognize (Boschma, 1999; Brush et al., 1999; Mortimer & McGann, 2005; Puzan, 2003; Shkimba & Flynn, 2005). Within the realities of health care in the latter half of the 20th century such constructions of nursing became increasingly challenged as the face of nursing in North America became (or was recognized as) more diverse (Brush et al., 1999). Because nurse historians participate in constructing historical knowledge in a particular way, we must ask ourselves, how critical are we about our interpretations? How do more recent historical insights influence the questions we ask in our historical research? Do more critical historical accounts actually make us rethink our historical questions?

Being involved as subjective beings in our work ultimately changes us as our assumptions are unsettled by the process of interpretation itself. Here we offer our own experiences as nurse historians to illustrate how questions of subjectivity and identity confront the work of nursing history. Our aim is not to provide answers, but rather to invite further questions and reflection on our situatedness as nurse historians.

In the narratives that follow, the three philosophical perspectives—post-structuralist, phenomenological, and epistemological—serve as analytic lenses to explore and question the multiple meanings of subjectivity in our own work. Each subjective account has elements of all three perspectives, but also emphasizes a particular perspective. That is, Boschma's reflection on her analysis of oral history interviews with families who experienced mental illness emphasizes a post-structuralist perspective; Grypma's reflection on her study of Canadian missionary work in China emphasizes a phenomenological perspective; and Melchior's reflection on her biographical research of Edna Auger emphasizes an epistemological perspective. In each narrative, we reflect on our identification as nurse historians and the ways in which we are called upon as nurses and researchers—by ourselves, by our subjects, and by our audiences.

ANALYZING AND CONTEXTUALIZING WHAT HAPPENS "IN THE MOMENT"

Boschma

How am I, as a nurse, involved in the construction of my stories? This question arose for me, when, in a sudden moment, I nearly burst into tears while presenting on my oral history interviews with families who experienced mental illness at a recent nursing history conference. I still remember the particular moment: I talked about a daughter who resisted framing her mother's past behavior as mental illness. The daughter did not think her mother had schizophrenia, rather, the daughter argued: "She was, she just was, she was a good person... a really good mom, really good mom... Yeah, she really was."

I had not been emotional about the phrase when I did the analysis of the transcripts and prepared for the presentation. So, what happened in this moment? Why suddenly these tears? The experience was profound enough that I felt the need to reflect on how I was involved as a subject in my own research: Whose voice was speaking here? Reflection on subject position is an important part of the research process in analysis of recorded interviewing (Rapley, 2004). Moreover, questions from the audience propelled me into further reflection on this particular moment. My response seemed to be one of compassion, but how was that compassion to be explained? Did the emotional reaction tell something about me I had not articulated in words? Identities are multiple, and hardly ever chosen, Gerda Lerner (1997) emphasizes. Who was I in this moment?

My immediate thought was: It is the researcher in me reacting to this data. That is, I foregrounded my identity as the researcher bringing her own self to the interview and interpretation, deeply moved by the daughter's compassion for her mother, moved about the deep commitment of the daughter to construct a counter narrative, to use Molly Andrews term (Andrews, 2002, 2004)—that is, to go against the grain of the dominant medical discourse, not wanting to see her mother as a pathological being, but normalizing the experience. I remember I said something to that degree to the audience: "Doesn't my emotion demonstrate my involvement as a subject too, co-constructing in the moment of interpretation?" One conference participant confirmed this perspective. She later commented, "I thought, wow, is this person enmeshed with her data." It made me think, was I? I pondered whether I was keeping the necessary distance that comes with an expert role. Or is it only through the intimacy of interpretation that the voice of the interviewee can be brought out? Is a certain level of emotional involvement unavoidable? A good thing perhaps? Or should such experience be framed as over-involvement? A risk of bias? As pointed out in the introduction, recent insights from qualitative social science and feminist theory have emphasized the situatedness of the researcher, challenging the idea of researcher neutrality or objectivity (Berger & Quinney, 2005; Gluck & Patai, 1991; Iacovetta, 1999; Seale, 2004). Personal involvement, I reassured myself, is a necessary, unavoidable, and valuable aspect of oral historiography.

How, then, was I involved as a subject? What identity did I (co-)construct? Another member of the audience catalyzed the question whether and how I constructed myself as a nurse (versus a researcher) in that moment: "How are you, as a nurse, involved in these interviews?" That question made me think about my subjectivity as a nurse in this project: Was my emotional response to the daughter's normalizing strategies in dealing with mental illness a reflection of my compassion as a nurse? Did my tears in the end reveal my identity as a nurse? To my surprise, I felt ambivalent about this thought. I wanted to argue that my tears did not reflect my identity as a nurse, but my "resistance" to being categorized as a "compassionate" nurse raised further self-doubt. Did I not want to be identified as a nurse? What was this ambivalence about? Upon reflection,

I concluded that my ambivalence could be best explained as a reaction in the moment to the experience of being categorized (Varcoe, 2006). I remember how I felt subjected, positioned as a nurse, and I was not sure what was meant by that categorization. What construction of *nurse* was at stake here? Was I a nurse who had become emotional and compassionate about her charge? What process of objectivation, in the words of Foucault, was going on? What meaning was bestowed upon me and, more importantly, did I want to be framed as a nurse in that *particular* way?

I wondered about the deeper meaning of the ambivalence I felt about being immediately categorized as a nurse. As pointed out earlier, nurses may resist the category with its implied and socially constructed meanings, but can't escape it. Compassion may be understood to be a natural characteristic of a nurse, but it is not: It is a construct, not an essence. The collective understanding of what it means to be a nurse reflects historical "baggage," which we have to confront, consciously, or unconsciously, the moment we are identified as being a nurse. Compassion of nurses is neither necessarily good nor inherent, revealing its situated, constructed nature. That is, in some situations being compassionate and emotional is seen as bad, unprofessional, or overinvolved—reflective of a gendered coding of human experiences as the typical feminine (over) emotional response. In other situations, compassion and tears can be perceived as reflecting a heroic identity such as the compassionate sufferer, the submissive but heroic helper, or the empathetic listener (Jones, 1988). Which of the images were being applied to me, if any? Even if I did not want to comply with being framed into either of these images, could I simply reject them as nonapplicable, arguing that my emotional response reflected something else? Probably not. As feminist analyses have clearly indicated, we cannot simply move away from the historical constructions we are caught up in (Riley, 1988).

Perhaps part of my struggle with accepting an interpretation of my compassionate response as reflective of my identity as a nurse comes, indirectly, from my identity and experience as a historian. As a nurse historian I am keenly aware that the gendered image of a nurse as *compassionate* (and female, and white, and middle class) is historically situated. In resisting the image of *me* as a compassionate nurse, I resist being framed as an emotional being in a particular way. I am ambivalent about the connection between *compassion* and *nurse*. Whereas I would like to embrace an image of empathetic nurses having a genuine interest in the patients (and their families) entrusted in their care, I would rather reject being seen as a feminine, overemotional, nonintellectual, if not irrational being—a stereotypical response nurses had to deal with in the past, not unlike women in general, and which still persists in contemporary images. I clearly resist being identified with such an image that took hold in a particular historical context. In the current context of nursing, any unquestioned connection between compassion and nursing (if in the stereotypical sense) no longer makes sense, if it ever did. In the second half of the 20th century, nurses have taken on more diverse roles and responsibilities and have more diverse backgrounds in terms of ethnicity, education, and gender, generating new questions about what it means to be a nurse.

Reflecting on my identity as a nurse (and my tears) forced me to think about questions of identity, subjectivity, and performance in (my) narrative analysis and interpretation (Chamberlayne, Bornat, & Wengraf, 2000). To better understand how my identity as a nurse influences the way I reconstruct lives in my analysis, I turn to the notion of nursing-as-performance. In performance theory, one's identity is not static, never a given, but a fluid going back and forth between the individual experience and the larger social context (Burke, 2005; Chamberlayne et al., 2000). Butler (1990) uses the metaphor of the enactment of a script to relate identity and performance. Valverde (1990), speaking from a post-structural perspective, argues "the fragmented, unstable subject [...] is not regarded as a rational autonomous unit producing meanings and values, but rather as being constituted in the ebb and flow of conflicting meanings generated by various discourses" (p. 228). Drawing on multiple identities, narratives, interpretations (as enacted stories), and biographies, *create* selfhood rather than reveal it (Rapley, 2004).

Which identities did I enact in creating my selfhood in that very moment that I became emotional? It was not until some further reflection after the conference and discussion with my colleagues that I realized that another identity was involved here, beyond, or in addition to, me being a researcher or a nurse. Perhaps neither the voice of a researcher nor the voice of the nurse ultimately may have triggered my emotional response. An *older* voice may have triggered my tears. That is, my personal roots, my own role in my family, and my identity as a daughter committed to see her mother as good came to speak here. As I now see it, I strongly identified with the story of the interviewee who persisted in seeing her mother as good. My construction as a compassionate nurse drew upon, or was intertwined with, an older identity of being a second daughter in the family, shaping my identity as a caretaker and a helper (Hargrave & Pfitzer, 2003; Kerr & Bowen, 1988). I strongly related to the action of the daughter in the interview, likely because I saw in her experience a reflection of my own.

My own experiences as a daughter, albeit in different circumstances and context, likely sensitized me to pick up on and respond to what I perceived to be the remarkable emotional work done by this daughter to support her mother and foreground her mother's strengths, resisting framing her as a dysfunctional or pathological being. How we bring our biography to the interview or to the interpretation is not predetermined, but happens in the moment of (self)-construction (Day Sclater, 2004; Rapley, 2004). I realized that the only way I could answer the question of how I as a nurse shape my interpretation was if I acknowledged some of the multiple identities involved—such as a researcher, a nurse, and a daughter. If I did not include this multiplicity of identities, I felt I would not do justice to who I was in that moment. Resistance, I now realize, may be provoked by the anticipation or feeling to be at risk, or to be "framed" in a unidimensional or essentialist interpretation that does not fully reflect who you experience yourself to be in that moment. The category of nurse just didn't explain it for me, at least not if it was understood in a limited or essentialist way. Moreover, another identity seemed more fundamental to my emotional response. I was hesitant about being "culturally coded" based on that moment of becoming emotional. I was hesitant to embrace the descriptor "compassionate nurse" because of the images it provoked *for me.* Acceptance of the category *nurse* comes with a deep awareness of the contested history of the category, something that is rooted in my identity as a historian and which probably makes me the "nurse historian" that I am. I can only resist any essentializing categorization of myself if I acknowledge the multiple, intersected identities involved—that is researcher, nurse, and daughter, in this particular case. In acknowledging my multiplicity, I also reconstruct or recreate how a nurse can be understood.

The notion of a nurse being a woman naturally equipped with female compassion is a historically constructed notion, which can be deconstructed, but also haunts us the minute we reproduce ourselves as nurses: We are situated in our past and context. It is not necessarily that I want to give up on the notion of compassion so much as to avoid any essentializing notions of *nurse.* Rather, we may seek to enact compassion in new ways, in my case, for example, in reflecting on my multiple identities as a woman/daughter, nurse, *and* researcher. Bringing these three identities together is possible today in a way that may have seemed impossible 100 years ago. Enactment, or performance, holds on to a sense of activism (renewal) while also exploring difference. If we, as nurses, want to continue to be constructed as beings of compassion, then we need to continue to explore both the historical roots of our compassion and the construction of compassion in our own individual acts. I believe it is the interconnectedness between our individual multiple identities, past and present, that work or produce us as certain beings in the moment, here and now. As Valverde (1990) puts it, none of our identities "exist in ontological, pre-discursive structures, but rather are constantly produced" (p. 235).

In the process of questioning what happened in that moment, a process that had multiple players involved, I became the subject of interpretation myself. Understanding how we draw from multiple identities in constructing ourselves as a certain being or certain interpreter may help us in doing historical analysis. If we reconstruct the life of a nurse, or of any person in the process of interpretation, we never should assume that only one identity is at stake. Nor should we frame the person in a one-dimensional or essentialist way. Susan Reverby (1999), in her careful analysis of the Tuskegee Syphilis Case, and especially of the role of Nurse Rivers, reminds us of this importance. She argues that Nurse Rivers' words *and her silence* reflect multiple "voices that allowed her to accommodate and resist the pressures of race, class, profession, and gender at the very same moment in differing and subtle ways" (p. 20). Reverby foregrounds Nurse Rivers' resistance rather than her compliance, which stood out in earlier portrayals. Doing justice to the subjectivity of a person requires exploring the multiplicity of identities and categories involved. If we seek to reach that level of complexity in our analysis, carefully listening to the multiple responses involved, including our own, we can deepen the historical understanding of the identities of the subjects involved in our work. In deep reflection on our interpretation, on who we are as nurses, women, daughters, researchers, and on the pressures we experience "to be in certain ways," we can resist, perform, rethink, and reframe taken for granted ideas about nursing and nurses. We may resist certain preconceived notions, such as being a "compassionate nurse," by seeing them as constructed ones, embedded in multiple identities we carry with us from our past experiences into every (day) ordinary life (Andrews, Day Sclater, Squire, & Tamboukou, 2004).

In reflection upon our multiple identities, we can come to critical understandings of the notion of *nurse*. In narration and in the interpretation of the stories we listen to, we (re)construct our identity as a nurse. In the interpretation, we can find or trace "evidence" of the nurse we have become. Our identity as a nurse is constructed from multiple (past) identities we bring toward what we seek and want nursing to be. Similarly, the compassion we bring to life as human beings has multiple roots, enacted and re-enacted in different contexts. It is in this process of reciprocity or interconnected subjectivities that our reactions and responses as nurses must be understood.

RECONSTRUCTING LIVES: WHOSE LIFE IS IT ANYWAYS?

Grypma

When I was 15, I decided I wanted to become a missionary nurse. Born to Dutch immigrant parents and reared in a conservative Christian

Reformed home, school, and church, my decision to attend a Mennonite Brethren boarding school in Saskatchewan for grades 11 and 12 was considered radical. Yet, my parents, somewhat courageously I think, acquiesced to this switch of religious and cultural allegiance. At age 15, then, I became immersed in a strange new culture—one that emphasized personal salvation, evangelism, and missionary service—and somehow I felt right at home. For the next 2 years I lived in dormitories with children of mostly Mennonite parents; some were children of missionaries living in exotic-sounding places such as Papua New Guinea and Zaire. I came to believe that missionary work was an inherently dangerous profession: The father of one of my schoolmates was kidnapped and brutally murdered in South America. The father of another died in Papua New Guinea. Although I was never attracted to the evangelistic aspect of missionary work—perhaps due more to my introverted disposition than any theological disagreement—I *was* attracted to the notion of living in what I imagined would be a multilingual, multicultural, serious-minded expatriate community in a foreign country. Nursing, then, was a ticket to international work.

I never did become a missionary nurse. Over the years, as I experienced life as a nurse in places such as Uganda, Kenya, Guyana, northern Canada, and China, I began to realize that missionary nursing as I perceived it does not exist. And I began to wonder if it ever really did.

In this section I approach the question, "How do we, as nurse historians, construct our stories?" with the premise that all writers bring their values and beliefs to their writing, consciously or not (Garrison, 1992). Historians recognize, I think, that subjectivity influences what *others* write (that is, the sources we are analyzing). For example, Nelson (2002) suggests that the challenge for contemporary historians is to understand the perspective of the authors of sources and the context in which those sources were produced. Nock (1991) similarly suggests that all historical evidence should be analyzed in terms of the motives and social positions of the authors. We acknowledge, then, how subjectivity affects the data we analyze, but pay less attention to how *our* subjectivity influences what *we* write. In researching nursing history, what difference does it make if the historian is, or is not, a nurse? How does our identity (our ethnicity, gender, race, class, nationality, profession, etc.) influence our analysis? More personally, how does my own lived experience as a Christian nurse specializing in intercultural work shape my interpretation of missionary nursing in China? How does *my* subjectivity influence what is revealed and what is concealed? As I explore these questions, my aim is not to provide definitive answers, but rather to bring to the surface some of the underlying tensions inherent in historiography; to call us to reflect on how what we bring to our work both benefits and detracts from our nursing subjects, and to stimulate discussion about ways we can bring balance to the yin and yang of objectivity and subjectivity.

Subjectivity and Historiography

> If the poem is the poet, the novel the novelist, and the picture the painter, is the biographer the biography?
>
> —Leon Edel, cited in Dee Garrison, 1992, p. 68

In the introduction to their book titled *The Challenge of Feminist Biography,* editors Alpern, Antler, Perry, and Scobie (1992) argue that objectivity is an illusion in historiography. Historians, they write, must give up "the arrogance of believing that we can, once and for all, get our foremothers right" (p. 11). There is no such thing as a "definitive" biography because new data might become available, and existing data are always open to reinterpretation. As Cameron (1991) has noted, two people with access to the same material would produce different versions of the same life. A single life may stimulate a variety of interpretations because each biographer approaches the data with a unique perspective or worldview, and therefore a unique set of questions. Our subjectivity as researchers—or the way we bring ourselves into our research—may explain why certain subjects, such as Florence Nightingale, stimulate a seemingly endless variety of biographies. Nightingale's letters, for example, may seem frozen in time, but the questions being asked of them are ever changing.

Garrison (1992) writes that a biographer's work is part detached scientific research, and part an autobiographical process. Responding to Edel's question: *If the poem is the poet, the novel the novelist, and the picture the painter, is the biographer the biography?* Garrison responds with an emphatic, *Yes.* Biographical interpretation, she writes, "reveals a peculiarly reciprocal relationship between author and subject. The biographer is visible in the selection of documents and testimony, in the intuitive choice of a quote or incident to move along the story and, above all, in the choice to write this particular life and not another" (p. 68). Rather than stifling or denying our subjectivity, feminist historians call us to be explicit about it and to be honest with ourselves about how our fears, desires, interests, and values might influence our renderings of our subjects. The challenge of the biographer is to produce a true—that is, accurate—portrait of a subject. In attempting to produce a true likeness, the biographer is caught between the need to adhere to facts and the need to interpret a subject (Halpenny, 1991). We approach the evidence with the intention of trying to understand not only facts (dates, times, places, events) but also the character of the person writing about those facts. And as we seek out the nature of our subjects in our studies, we reveal our own.

Subjectivity and the Study of Missionary Nurses

"I collect rivers" wrote Ethel Johns in an editorial to the *Canadian Nurse* journal in the 1930s. Johns was reminiscing about her work in Europe with the Rockefeller Foundation. Specifically, she was reminiscing about the Danube and other rivers around the world to which she was drawn and from which she drew strength, even on recollection. In a similar way, I collect living rooms. To be invited into someone's living room, particularly in an unfamiliar country or culture, is to me a sacred and intimate invitation to the very heart of a person and their family. At age 17, I sat in the formal living room of distant relatives in Holland, looking through lace curtains to a family-owned hardware store a few meters across the dijk while we attempted to converse with our Dutch/English dictionaries on our laps. Nurses are routinely invited into homes during crises and milestones, a privilege of our work. At age 22, I sat in the living room of a Tsimshian woman on a remote First Nations island where I worked as an outpost nurse. I was perched beside her on the edge of her couch, taking her blood pressure as relatives lined the walls, observing, having summoned me to help with her severe headache. Suddenly her left arm and leg jerked, and she slipped into unconsciousness in front of us—the result, we later found out, of a brain aneurysm. At age 23, I knelt on a straw mat in the dark, one-room hut of a Ugandan mother who had been hemorrhaging since her baby's birth 9 days earlier, and I listened to her gurgling lungs with my stethoscope as her family stood in the shadows around us. And last fall, I sat in the receiving room of an 84-year-old Chinese nurse in Kaifeng, China, the only surviving nurse of the class of 1942, perhaps the only Chinese nurse left in Henan province who was taught by Canadian missionary nurses. We sat together on a couch with her four children and a group of onlookers as I showed her a DVD on my laptop—a DVD I had made and had translated into Mandarin about the history—her history—of Canadian nurses in Henan between 1888 and 1947.

When I approach data related to the history of missionary nurses in China—most recently of Canadian nurses interned under the Japanese there—I do so with a recognition that my position as a researcher, not unlike my position as a nurse, privileges me to enter the metaphorical living room—the most private space, a sacred space—of my subjects. I am always the nurse—observing, interpreting, reassuring, and, above all, careful not to harm my subjects and their families in my writing. As in my intercultural nursing practice, I tend to conceal my own responses to my encounters with my subjects, not admitting how my own values, beliefs, and assumptions are challenged, altered, affirmed, or denied as a result of my ongoing contact with missionary nurses through their surviving papers, photos, artifacts, and family members—that is, how deep encounters with my subjects transform me, and how I need it to be so. For example, Canadian nurse Betty Gale's journal from a Japanese internment camp in 1942 affirms Victor Frankl's assertion that one can find joy in a place of confinement and suffering (Frankl, 1984/1946), and yet, when I travel with Betty's daughter to Shanghai and stand in Pudong district, the area where the family was interned, and she shows me the scar on her hand from an incident described by her mother in her camp diary 60 years ago, I wonder how much of her mother's writing involved self-censorship. The daughter's scar came from grabbing an exposed hot water pipe in the camp. Betty writes of her anxiety over her daughters burned hand, but does not express anger or frustration at the situation, only gratefulness for any help received. I wonder whether her joy-in-suffering discourse, the same joy-in-suffering discourse I've always heard in relation to missionary work, is truth—is completely honest. Is Betty self-censoring for the benefit of her captors, for her daughter (to whom she dedicated the journal), for herself?

I self-censor, too, I've come to realize, and this brings problems of its own. I resist being forthright about my religious identity in my writing—partly because I do not want readers to make any assumptions about my stance on particular issues, and partly because my beliefs are a work in progress. What has been most surprising to me has been when readers suggest that I am unsympathetic toward missionaries, or anti-Christian, in fact. A reader of one article I wrote took my criticism of missionary work to mean that I was intolerant of religious aspirations. The reviewer of another stated that I presented myself as a "progressive secularist," interested in but not necessarily appreciative of the religious aspect of missionary nursing. By self-censoring, do I censor my subjects?

Whether or not I choose to recognize it, my religious identity impacts my work. So does my professional identity as a nurse, but for different reasons. Recently a non-nurse reviewer commented on my lack of description about nursing practice and education in a manuscript I had submitted for publication. As a nurse writing mostly to nursing audiences, I was shocked to realize how much I overlooked, and therefore obscured, what I knew well. I was grateful for the comment because once this was pointed out to me it was relatively easy to remedy the situation. It is not that I do not know nursing well enough; it is that I know it *too* well. Sometimes what is missing in our writing, and in the data we review, is that which is taken for granted. How do we, as nurses, construct our stories? Consciously or not, we bring our values and experiences to our writing, and, consciously or not, a bit of ourselves is revealed in everything we write.

THE SUBJECTIVE POSITION OF THE BIOGRAPHER

Melchior

Ever since conducting my doctoral research I have been intrigued by the life of Edna Auger (1876–1932), a graduate of Medicine Hat General Hospital (MHGH) located in Medicine Hat, in the southeastern area in the province of Alberta, Canada. She worked as an operating room nurse, educator, and nursing superintendent, and she was a recipient of the Royal Red Cross for her service in WWI (Melchior, 2005). I could not resist the temptation to write a biography on her.

I realized, however, that constructing an adequate and accurate biographical picture of Auger would be difficult because of limited sources, especially unofficial ones that often contain a more personal record. I was inspired by Sonya Grypma's (2005) delineation of critical issues in biography—"addressing worthiness in subject selection...addressing limited sources in data collection...addressing truth in data analysis" (pp. 173–178). I believed wholeheartedly that my subject was worthy of the effort.

Thus, my biography begins with interpretation because, first: "Why do I believe that Edna Auger is a worthy subject?" and second: "What is it that leads me to fascination about her career rather than another?" There were other notable nurses from the school who emerged from my doctoral research—for example, Victoria Winslow who was the first president of the Alberta Association of Registered Nurses (AARN), Elizabeth MacDougall who also won the Royal Red Cross in WWI, and Mary Rowles. Rowles was the founder of the school's year book and alumni association, a student of post-graduate work at McGill, a nursing superintendent in British Columbia, and actively professional throughout her life. Yet, they did not capture my interest in the same way.

Grypma (2005) also notes, biography in nursing is sparse, and perhaps mirrors the gendered bias toward women in the workforce. Most biographies that do exist are about *great* nurses; however, there is also a need for biographical research about *ordinary* nurses: What was their experience? What were their perceptions of their education and the working world of nursing? I had not specifically considered whether Edna Auger would fit into either the great or ordinary category. But, I did want to understand her life more fully, and in some way restore her to a rightful place in nursing history, at least in the regional history of Medicine Hat and Alberta. The "lost" women, as Alpern et al. (1992) argue, do not fit the masculine biographical template. In Medicine Hat there are no streets or bridges named after Auger—that privilege has been reserved for men of influence in commerce and politics. In addition, the Auger family fonds list Edna as a daughter of the family, but no mention is made of her achievements. Marriages by other daughters, however, are recorded—illustrating the "marriage plot" as the defining feature of notable female success (Alpern et al., 1992, p. 9).

Obviously, I do believe that Auger achieved some kind of greatness. And possibly that greatness stemmed from her unique nursing life. As I recounted her experiences, which I will touch on here, I knew that I was intrigued by a professional journey that mixed skilled practice with determined leadership in a variety of contexts.

Edna Mabel Auger was born in Chatham, Ontario, in 1876. Her family moved to Maple Creek in southwestern Saskatchewan when she was 7, and where she received her early schooling. She returned to Ontario for a high school education. Auger entered the MHGH School of Nursing in 1903 at the age of 27. After graduating in 1906, she worked at MHGH as the operating room (OR) supervisor before traveling to New York for further education and OR work in a private hospital. She returned to Medicine Hat in 1912 to take up the position of assistant lady superintendent. In April 1915, Auger went overseas with the Number One Canadian General Hospital Corps (Melchior, 2004). She spent most of the next 3 years in the war zone and received the Royal Red Cross in 1918 for "valuable services with the Armies in France and Flanders" (Richardson, 2000, pp. 5–6). Her valuable services included staying with her patients at a front-line nursing station when it was bombed; she was later dug out of the rubble. On her return to Canada in the fall of 1919, she rested at home in Maple Creek "until the summer of 1920 then went north to organize a hospital at Grande Prairie" (Obituary, *Medicine Hat News*, 1932, p. 5). She applied for and was successful in obtaining the position of nursing superintendent at MHGH in the spring of 1922; there were seven other qualified applicants from across North America. In May of 1932, Auger died, possibly from kidney failure, 1 month after returning home from an AARN meeting in Edmonton (Melchior, 2005).

During her tenure as nursing superintendent in Medicine Hat, Auger was active with the AARN as chair of the finance committee and convener for the committee on the minimum curriculum for training schools in the province of Alberta. She marked the obstetrical papers for Alberta's registration examinations from 1922 until her death in 1932. She was also the AARN's representative to the Weir Report—an influential national survey of nursing education used as a blueprint for improving nursing education in Canada; it was published in 1932 (Melchior, 2004).

Interestingly, Auger's leadership in Medicine Hat was marked by several power struggles: with the male secretary–treasurer of the hospital; with the Women's Hospital Aid Society [WHAS]; and with one group of graduated nurses. In all, she appears to have garnered support both from the Board and eventually from the WHAS. But it is the conflict between Auger and her staff that is the most enigmatic. On May 20, 1924, a special committee of the Board was struck to "investigate certain charges made by certain members of the staff in the discipline of the hospital" (MHGH, 1924a). In June, 2 years after Auger assumed the position of superintendent, all the graduated nurses on staff filed their resignations. The board asked them to reconsider, but they replied: "that it was impossible for them to reconsider their resignations; the question of harmony between the nurses and their Superintendent could not be brought about" (MHGH, 1924b). In July, there was a request from the resigned nurses for a month's pay in lieu of holidays—"claim they were entitled." The request was not granted (MHGH, 1924c).

Beyond a concern about discipline, no other explanations for the resignations were recorded in the minutes of the board. So, what can be discerned from the evidence? There had been a decrease in the number of graduated staff because of budget cuts, but this was beyond Auger's control. There was a dramatic rise in illness following the reduction in staff, and the deaths of two nursing students. But again, this was beyond Auger's control. Within her control, she had made constructive recommendations to the board that were implemented. For example, her recommendations included: a diet kitchen on the top floor of the hospital to save nurses running up and down the stairs; to increase the OR supervisor's wages; then later, increases for the other supervisors, and a new sterilizer for the OR. The evidence suggests that disharmony began after the new "Rules and Regulations for Nurses" were introduced by Auger in late 1922. There had not previously existed a rule book, and "reading between the lines" it is likely that graduated nurses considered themselves demeaned by such policies as a "sick parade" (MHGH, n.d.).

As McGinnis argues (1992), "the biographer is like a detective" trying to figure out not only what has occurred but also why it has occurred (p. 45). Remaining neutral or objective is probably impossible. I would not be conducting this biography if there was not a fascination with the subject, so neutrality is not a reasonable possibility. But, I do have a responsibility to attempt an interpretation that includes as many "sides" as possible. Unlike a biographer from another discipline, my interpretation of the questions "what and why" is colored by my experiences as a nurse, which might lead me to the other sides of the story. And, my experience tells me that something more personal than working hours or assigned duties had offended the graduated staff. It is likely that Auger had assumed a more regimented style of administration following her stint in the war, and the book of rules and regulation would attest to that. I know from experience that new policies implemented quickly by a new supervisor, which do not take into account the professional standards that nurses acquire through the socializing process of education, are often met with resistance. This resistance, leading possibly to insubordination, had been brewing for awhile. Perhaps, if the rules and regulations had applied only to nursing students, rather than including graduate staff, the "revolt" may not have happened.

I now address my question about why Auger has caught my interest. First, I think that Auger demonstrated an ability to straddle both worlds of practice and leadership. She had a clear understanding of nursing and leadership in the workplace, as I have outlined earlier, yet, she also had influence with the AARN and in national and international professional bodies. I believe that it is nurses like Auger who are needed to mend the rift that developed and still exists between the rank-and-file and nursing leadership. How to mend that rift is a concern of mine, and one that I have addressed in other papers.

Secondly, I envy Auger's opportunity to participate in a watershed event such as WWI. I often think that some of the great events have passed me by, although conversely I am afraid of being involved in something so horrendous. Living vicariously through Auger is safer, but of course less exciting.

Our perceived notion about the excitement of war-time nursing also requires reflection. The excitement and wonder might arise from the diaries, notes, and stories left by military nurses who recorded memorable moments and events. But, what is exciting about wounds, death, disease, and dirt? As Mann (2000) introduces Clare Gass's War Diary, she notes that the "more routine her days, the less she commented" (p. xi). The time between diary entries must have been spent performing a multitude of tasks including emptying bedpans and urinals, "making and equipping beds to obtaining stores from the central supply, stocking the tiny ward kitchen, and arranging space for the charge nurse to make her report"(p. xxix). Besides changing dressings for combat wounds and dealing with the madness of "shell shock," the duties are not that different from normal hospital routine of the time—except for the conditions and the setting. And the conditions were not glamorous. The "boys" who came in from the trenches were "dirty, bloody, and lousy" (p. xxxi). Yes, the nursing work was invaluable and appreciated by the "boys," but did the excitement of caring for the wounded actually outweigh the hardship and drudgery of the everyday?

As I ponder further, I wonder, has something else driven this research? As Grypma quotes Leon Edel: "Is the biographer the biography?"(noted by Grypma earlier in this chapter). Like Auger, I straddle a world between clinical practice and leadership and try to find a balance between the two. While my first loyalty has been to supporting front-line practice, I endeavor to foster acknowledgment and respect for the work of both. After our presentation on subjectivity and interpretation, some conference participants commented that I have a physical resemblance to Auger. This startled me, but it led me to rethink my reasons for researching the life and work of this nurse. Have I found someone in the past who reflects my dilemma and position in the present day?

CONCLUSION

We agree with Chandler's (2005) observation that "subjectivity—both our subject's and our own—shapes the content and interpretation of our work" (p. 48). Although Chandler was addressing oral historians, it is clear that subjectivity is inherent in all historiography. By reflecting on and trying to articulate our own subjectivity as nurse historians, we have discovered ways in which post-structuralist, phenomenological, and epistemological perspectives influence our work. In her reflection on her experience presenting data from oral history interviews, Geertje Boschma grapples with the post-structuralist question: "What does it mean to be *categorized* as 'nurse'?" By struggling to identify the underlying cause of her unexpected emotional reaction to the words of a daughter recorded in an oral interview, Boschma resists being interpreted or objectified in a *particular* way. In recognizing her own ambivalence toward being identified as a nurse, Boschma realizes that it is her subjectivity as a historian that refutes the automatic association between "compassion" and "nursing": Compassion, she argues, is a contested and socially constructed notion that situates contemporary nursing (and contemporary nurses like Boschma) in its historic (gendered, racialized) past. On deeper reflection, Boschma traces her subjective response to her data to her identity as a daughter. She concludes that subjectivity in her case involves multiple identities (daughter/woman, nurse, and historian), each of which influences and shapes the other. And each of which ultimately influences her choices and emphases in her historical work.

In her reflection on her role as a nurse historian in her work on missionary nurses in China, Sonya Grypma explores how her subjectivity as a Christian nurse with an interest in intercultural clinical practice might influence her historical research. Grypma especially grapples with the phenomenological question: "How do our experiences as nurses 'carry over' into our historical interpretations?" She concludes that her religious, cultural, and professional selves naturally permeate her research—at times assisting her to "see" things perhaps otherwise invisible, but at other times "blinding" her toward areas that she might take for granted. Being a nurse, particularly one who has routinely adapted her work to the intimate and varied living spaces of culturally diverse patients and clients, helps her to feel at home in the intimacy of biography—of people's narratives. Attuned to both what is said/seen and what is silent/hidden, Grypma reflects on the relationship between (the researcher's) lived experience and subjectivity. She believes that her identity as a nurse subconsciously influences her historiographic decisions and opportunities. Yet, while accepting that the biography is necessarily a reflection of the biographer, Grypma rejects the notion that researchers may disregard objectivity. Rather, historians must strive for a balance between objectivity and subjectivity—recognizing that if the former represents rigor toward the subject, the latter represents relationship with it.

Finally, in her reflection on her desire to research Edna Auger, Florence Melchior attends the epistemological question: "How are we positioned as 'knowers' in our interpretation?" As Melchior reflects on why she is drawn to Auger's life, she asks herself why Auger and not another? What is it about Auger's life that makes her a subject worthy of historiographic analysis? She addresses laudable aspects of Auger's life, her ambition and accomplishments in the midst of oppressive hierarchical structures. She finds herself envious of Auger's wartime adventures, and vicariously enjoys the drama recollected in her memoirs. Yet, there is something beneath the surface of Auger's life that is not immediately accessible to the researcher. Existing documents hint at the certain frustrations, dissentions, and personality conflicts, and the vagueness piques Melchior's curiosity. After all, conflict and drama adds life and character—and interest—to the human story. It is here that Melchior draws on her subjective experience as a nurse to peek under the carpet, as it were, to try to understand gaps in the data related to the mass resignation of graduated nurses while Auger was a superintendent. Melchior suggests that the resignations were simply the boiling-over point of a power struggle simmering for awhile. Specifically, the resignations represented a resistance to Auger's misdirected and perhaps insensitive display of authority.

In our individual historiographic projects, our subjectivity as nurses, historians, and women necessarily influence our work. We bring our cultural, religious, professional, familial, and gendered selves—that is, our multiple identities—to our research. These identities act as lenses through which we interpret the world—in some cases distorting our subjects, while in others, bringing them into sharper focus.

REFERENCES

Alpern, S., Antler, J., Perry, E. I., & Scobie, I. W. (Eds.). (1992). *The challenge of feminist biography: Writing the lives of modern American women.* Chicago: University of Illinois Press.

Andrews, M. (2002). Memories of mother: Narrative reconstructions of early maternal influence. *Narrative Inquiry, 12*(1), 1–6.

Andrews, M. (2004). Living counter-narratives. In C. Seale, G. Gobo, J. F. Gubrium, & D. Silverman (Eds.), *Qualitative research practice* (pp. 109–112). Thousand Oaks, CA: Sage.

Andrews, M., Day Sclater, S., Squire, C., & Tamboukou, M. (2004). Narrative research. In C. Seale, G. Gobo, J. F. Gubrium, & D. Silverman (Eds.), *Qualitative research practice* (pp. 109–124). Thousand Oaks, CA: Sage.

Berger, R. J., & Quinney, R. (2005). The narrative turn in social inquiry. In R. J. Berger & R. Quinney (Eds.), *Storytelling sociology: Narrative as social inquiry* (pp. 13–16). Boulder, CO: Lynne Rienner Publishers.

Boschma, G. (1999). The gender specific role of male nurses in Dutch asylums. *International History of Nursing Journal, 4*(3), 13–19.

Burke, P. (2001). Overture. The new history: Its past and its future. In P. Burke (Ed.), *New perspectives on historical writing* (2nd ed., pp. 1–24). Cambridge, UK: Polity Press.

Burke, P. (2005). Performing history: The importance of occasions. *Rethinking History, 9*(1), 35–52.

Butler, J. (1990). Performative acts and gender constitution: An essay in phenomenology and feminist theory. In S. E. Case (Ed.), *Performing feminisms: Feminist critical theory and theatre* (pp. 270–282). Baltimore: John Hopkins University Press.

Brush, B. L., Lynaugh, J. E., Boschma, G., Rafferty, A. M., Stuart, M., & Tomes, N. J. (1999). *Nurses of all nations: A history of the International Council of Nurses, 1899–1999.* Philadelphia: Lippincott/Raven.

Cameron, E. (1991). Truth in biography. In R. B. Fleming (Ed.), *Boswell's children: The art of the biographer* (pp. 27–32). Toronto: Dundurn Press.

Chamberlayne, P., Bornat, J., & Wengraf, T. (Eds.). (2000). *The turn to biographical methods in social science: Comparative issues and examples.* London: Routledge.

Chandler, S. (2005). Oral history across generations: Age, generational identity and oral testimony. *Oral History, 33*(2), 48–56.

D'Antonio, P. (2006). History for a practice profession. *Nursing Inquiry, 13*(4), 242–248.

Davis, C. (1995). *Gender and the professional predicament in nursing.* Buckingham, UK: Open University Press.

Day Sclater, S. (2004). Narrative and subjectivity. In C. Seale, G. Gobo, J. F. Gubrium, & D. Silverman (Eds.), *Qualitative research practice* (pp. 112–115). Thousand Oaks, CA: Sage.

Dreyfus, H. L., & Rabinow, P. (1982). *Michel Foucault. Beyond structuralism and hermeneutics.* Chicago: University of Chicago Press.

Frankenberg, R. (1993). *White women, race matters: The social construction of whiteness.* Minneapolis: University of Minnesota Press.

Frankl, V. E. (1984). *Man's search for meaning.* New York: Pocket Books. (Original work published 1946)

Garrison, D. (1992). Two roads taken: Writing the biography of Mary Heaton Vorse. In S. Alpern, J. Antler, E. I. Perry, & I. W. Scobie (Eds.), *The challenge of feminist biography: Writing the lives of modern American women* (pp. 65–78). Chicago: University of Illinois Press.

Gluck, S. B., & Patai, D. (Eds.). (1991). *Women's words: The feminist practice of oral history.* New York: Routledge.

Grypma, S. (2005). Critical issues in the use of biographic methods in nursing history. *Nursing History Review, 13,* 171–187.

Halpenny, F. (1991). Expectations of biography. In R. B. Fleming (Ed.), *Boswell's children: The art of the biographer* (pp. 3–26). Toronto: Dundurn Press.

Harding, S. (2001). After absolute neutrality: Expanding "science." In M. Mayberry, B. Subramaniam, & L. H. Weasel (Eds.), *Feminist science studies* (pp. 291–304). London: Routledge.

Hargrave, T. D., & Pfitzer, F. (2003). *The new contextual therapy: Guiding the power of give and take.* New York: Brunner-Routledge.

Iacovetta, F. (1999). Post-modern ethnography, historical materialism, and decentering the (male) authorial voice: A feminist conversation. *Histoire Social/Social History, 32*(64), 275–293.

Jones, A. H. (Ed.). (1988). *Images of nurses: Perspectives from history, art, and literature.* Philadelphia: University of Pennsylvania Press.

Kerr, M., & Bowen, M. (1988). *Family evaluation: An approach based on Bowen theory.* New York: W. W. Norton & Company.

Lerner, G. (1997). *Why history matters: Life and thought.* Oxford: Oxford University Press.

Mann, S. (Ed.). (2000). *The war diary of Clare Glass, 1915–1918.* Montreal and Kingston: McGill-Queen's University Press.

McGinnis, J. D. (1992). Aimee Semple McPherson: Fantasizing the fantasizer? Telling the tale of a tale-teller. In R. B. Fleming (Ed.), *Boswell's children* (pp. 45–56). Toronto and Oxford: Dundurn Press.

Medicine Hat General Hospital. (n.d.). *Training School for Nurses at the Medicine Hat General Hospital: Rules and Regulations.* Medicine Hat, AB, Canada: Author.

Medicine Hat General Hospital. (1924a, May 20). *Minutes of the Board.* Esplanade Archives. Medicine Hat, AB, Canada: M86.28.2.

Medicine Hat General Hospital. (1924b, June 2). *Minutes of the Board.* Esplanade Archives. Medicine Hat, AB, Canada: M86.28.2.

Medicine Hat General Hospital. (1924c, June 9). *Minutes of the Board.* Esplanade Archives. Medicine Hat, AB, Canada: M86.28.2.

Melchior, F. (2004). *Nursing student labour, education, and patient care at the Medicine Hat General Hospital, 1890–1930.* Unpublished doctoral thesis, University of Calgary, Calgary, Alberta, Canada.

Melchior, F. (2005). Edna Mabel Auger, 1876–1932. *AlbertaRN, 61*(10), 13–14.

Mol, A. (2006). Proving or improving: On health care research as a form of self-reflection. *Qualitative Health Research, 16*(3), 405–414.

Mortimer, B., & McGann, S. (Eds.). (2005). *New directions in the history of nursing.* London: Routledge Taylor & Francis Group.

Nelson, S. (2002). The fork in the road: Nursing history vs. the history of nursing? *Nursing History Review, 10,* 175–188.

Nock, D. A. (1991). Biographical truth. In R. B. Fleming (Ed.), *Boswell's children: The art of the biographer* (pp. 33–39). Toronto: Dundurn Press.

Obituary. (1932, May 5). Edna Mabel Auger. *Medicine Hat News,* p. 5.

Puzan, E. (2003). The unbearable whiteness of being (in nursing). *Nursing Inquiry, 10*(3), 193–200.

Rapley, T. (2004). Interviews. In C. Seale, G. Gobo, J. F. Gubrium, & D. Silverman (Eds.), *Qualitative research practice* (pp. 15–33). Thousand Oaks, CA: Sage.

Reinharz, S. (1997). Who am I? The need for a variety of selves in the field. In R. Herz (Ed.), *Reflexivity & VOICE* (pp. 3–20). Thousand Oaks, CA: Sage.

Reverby, S. M. (1999). Rethinking the Tuskegee syphilis study: Nurse Rivers, silence and the meaning of treatment. *Nursing History Review, 7,* 3–28.

Richardson, S. (2000). Edna Mabel Auger, 1876–1932. In V. L. Bullough & L. Sentz (Eds.), *American nursing: A biographical dictionary* (pp. 5–6). New York: Springer Publishing.

Riley, D. (1988). *"Am I That Name?": Feminism and the category of "women" in history.* Minneapolis: University of Minnesota Press.

Roediger, D. R. (1999). *The wages of whiteness: Race and the making of the American working class* (rev. ed.). London: Verso.

Seale, C. (2004). Quality in qualitative research. In C. Seale, G. Gobo, J. F. Gubrium, & D. Silverman (Eds.), *Qualitative research practice* (pp. 409–419). Thousand Oaks, CA: Sage.

Shkimba, M., & Flynn, K. (2005). "In England we did nursing": Caribbean and British nurses in Great Britain and Canada, 1950–1970. In B. Mortimer & S. McGann (Eds.), *New directions in the history of nursing* (pp. 141–157). London: Routledge Taylor & Francis Group.

Sol, R. C. (1995). Subjectivity. In T. Honderich (Ed.), *The Oxford companion to philosophy* (p. 857). Oxford: Oxford University Press.

Valverde, M. (1990). Poststructuralist gender historians: Are we those names? *Labour/Le-Travail, 25,* 227–236.

Varcoe, C. (2006, December). *Interrogating the research process: Relational positionality and engaging difference.* Paper presented at the UBC School of Nursing Culture, Gender and Health Research Unit's second annual workshop, Vancouver, BC.

Wall, B. M. (2006). Textual analysis as a method for historians of nursing. *Nursing History Review, 14,* 227–242.

CHAPTER EIGHT

Historical Research in Developing Countries

Eleanor Krohn Herrmann

Conducting historical research in a developing country requires the same adherence to the rigors of historiography as is expected in an industrialized nation. Nursing's professional literature, however, has little information about how to address the intricacies and nuances related to the *process* of carrying out historical research in developing countries. While it is recognized that each developing country is unique, there are some considerations that are common to all (Masson, 1981). This chapter presents factors that should be considered in that process. It also provides related examples and rationale. The information, which is presented in three categories—preliminary work, in-country work, and home work—is based on the writer's collective experience in Central and South America and her experience as a practitioner of nursing, consultant, and nurse historian.

PRELIMINARY WORK

Recall what motivated you to consider undertaking historical research in a developing country. Was it your experience in the Peace Corps? A connection with your family's heritage? Your desire to become more culturally sensitive? Or some other trigger? Understanding your motivation can help provide the insight necessary to identify possible research questions and a framework for your investigation, as well as how to focus your study and delineate its parameters. Later, that introspection will be useful as you grapple with questions about how to handle contextual data and how to deal with variables.

Most critical at the outset is becoming familiar with the literature about the selected country. That should include social, political, health-related, educational, environmental, and economic views (D'Avanzo & Geissler, 2003). In addition to building a foundation of knowledge about the country, you will become aware of what data is, or is not, available in your home country thereby saving you time when in the developing country. It will also alert you to "holes" in the data that will need attention when you are out of your home country. Potential challenges may be a lack of knowledge about, or appreciation of, a developing country's own nursing history, as well as the lack of locally prepared historians, let alone nurse historians.

Because you will be a foreigner in the developing country, it should not be surprising that your motives for being there might come under suspicion. It is therefore wise to have a respected national of the country as an advocate who can vouch for your credibility and who can introduce you to relevant contacts. The national advocate can help identify potential candidates for oral history interviews and help allay any hesitation, skepticism, or distrust about the interview process. The advocate can also be helpful when you hope to use official documents and need official permission to do so. A caution is called for here. This researcher had received written approval at the ministerial level for such use, but was denied access by an underling who had the actual physical control of the documents. The reason for withholding the documents was unclear at the time, but to avoid antagonism and a possible ripple effect, the matter was "put on hold." Fortunately, another reliable source was later found. Had that not happened, the omission would likely have significantly influenced the findings of the study.

To facilitate the contemplated work in the developing country, it is prudent to avoid making assumptions about the availability of certain items. Find out, for example, if a copy machine is available. Answer: Yes. Cost is one dollar per page. Can I handle, turn over, or pick up an old document rotting from mildew or the moisture from a leaking roof or past hurricane, or must I photograph it to preserve its content? Is an Internet connection possible? Answer: Yes, if you walk a mile to reach a computer and then wait in line for your turn while five other people finish their business. Is there a secure work space where one can write and then leave their notes while pursuing further data? Yes, to the availability of a jerry-built carrel, but security is "at your own risk." And what about a quiet place to ponder, reflect, and cogitate about your findings? Answer: A hotel room, a friend's house, and a convent were all used by this writer, although the caged parrots in the friend's house were quite noisy, and the frequency of the bells in the convent were distracting. At the convent, the food provided by the nuns was so sparse that a perceived scandal was risked by this writer sneaking over the convent wall late at night to buy candy bars at a nearby bodega.

Some final words about preparation for your stay in a developing country. You need to stay healthy while you are there collecting your research data. However, such things as climate, insects, food, water, altitude, and lack of sleep can quickly change that situation, and as Bryant (1969) has warned in his classic book titled *Health in the Developing World,* "in most countries, unfortunately, health care is seriously inadequate" (p. xi). To compensate for that shortcoming, you may want to consider taking along some incidental over-the-counter supplies and drugs, such as Band-Aids and medications for gastrointestinal and respiratory problems. If, however, you get bitten by a snake, such as one called a Jumping Viper, ignore the foregoing and get to a local shaman or witch doctor ASAP! Alternative medicine may be appropriate for many health problems that arise in a foreign setting. For example, if you eat poisoned barracuda, the local cure is a broth made from its bones.

Another caveat: Develop a time schedule that you believe will allow you to fulfill your research plans...and then revise it allowing time for the unexpected. Examples of the unexpected include such things as the need to check an incomplete or missing citation, a request for a follow-up visit by an oral history interviewee, and even the threat of a hurricane.

IN-COUNTRY WORK

There is no "right way" to start looking for the in-country data for your study, but because you likely will have talked with someone about the available sources, it seems appropriate to discuss language and historical research methodology. Hopefully the researcher will speak and read the major language of the country in which the research will be conducted. The ability to comprehend the written word is particularly important because so much of historical research depends on written documents. If the researcher is limited to English in a non–English-speaking country, it is likely that communications will be reduced to exchanges with individuals who have had more opportunities in life than the general public (Masson, 1981). That disparity will limit the data and influence the findings of the research.

Using a competent translator is one way of addressing the problem. However, that slows the rate of communication, can be costly for the researcher, and can result in inaccuracies if the translator is not completely familiar with technical and nursing terminology. A better solution, although a long-term one, would be to return to the once-common

TABLE 8.1 Dealing With the Search for Data

Status (p = pending; d = done)	Sources to Be Explored	Notes
Government	Minister of Health	National plans; Colonial records; Archives; Libraries
	Chief Nursing Officer	Records of the School of Nursing (SON), status of nursing; Plans? Deadlines?
Ecclesiastic	Churches x five; Temples x one;	See Father John for Latin translation
	Convent	Order? Community activity?
	Mission Society	Goals & activities?
Nursing Education	SON faculty, Chief Nursing Officer	Achievements? Problems? Plans? Pictures? Graduate Study?
International Nursing	Chief Nursing Officer; SON Faculty; Health Ministry	Results of Caribbean & Latin reviews? Impact?
Newspapers	Editors, all national papers	Publicity for nursing? Street named to honor nurse
Individual Contacts	Older nurses; their descendants	Oral history on tape

requirement that all doctoral candidates have a working knowledge of at least one other modern language.

A decision about where you should start looking for the data for your research study is generally based on where you think you might get the greatest yield in relation to your research questions. The starting point may also simply be driven by serendipity or an uncanny feeling, or perhaps because your in-country advocate suggested it, or because the repository was closest to where you were living. At any rate, it really does not matter where you start because you will eventually investigate all the known sources to determine their value and appropriateness for your research. What is important is having a system to ensure that all the possible sources are indeed explored. A further benefit is that it can save time and energy, as well as the cost of having to make an additional international trip in the future. As an example, Table 8.1 reflects one way of dealing with the search for data that this author used in her research.

The first column lists the overall areas that you believe might hold information pertaining to the study and therefore should be investigated. Of note is the fact that all of the areas correspond to your preparatory reading. The "p" and the "d" key is a way to note your progress. The middle column contains potential sources for information while the right hand "Notes" column reminds you of specific topics that you want to pursue and questions that arise. All areas can be expanded periodically. Keeping the information in a spiral-bound notebook makes it easy to carry the information around, while simultaneously avoiding loose papers that could become a breach in confidentiality. A laptop or another method for recording data may also work, but you need to be sure that they are viable solutions in a developing country. Remember, that a power source may be intermittent, and you may not have the correct current to run a laptop in a developing country.

Networking during the in-country work period is a very effective tool, especially if you have gained the confidence of the people. The contacts that are made can lead to previously unknown caches of personal papers that have just been sitting there until someone like you comes along. One nurse told this writer, "I don't think they [the papers] are very important to anyone else, but I just couldn't part with them. I don't know what they [her family] will do with them when I'm gone." Now she knows; they will become part of a national archival collection. The content of the papers? They contained stories of her battle with diabetes in the late 1920s, before the time when insulin was generally available in a developing country. One value of the stories lies in the fact that such primary source data sometimes are the only corroborating evidence available. Networking was the other value; it was the means for bringing the stories to light.

In a developing country, more attention is generally given to the present and future than to the past. That outlook has contributed to difficulties the historian is likely to encounter—deteriorated buildings, documents riddled with book worms and other such creatures, and the absence of a climate-controlled central archival repository, to name a few. However these very conditions make developing countries fertile grounds for historical research, which is needed immediately for preservation.

HOMEWORK

After spending an extended period of time in a developing country, deeply immersed in historical research and study, it would not be unusual for a person to experience culture shock upon returning to their home country. Some extra sleep helps, but a magic elixir may also be music—such as a merengue from the Dominican Republic, calypso from Jamaica, or a steel-drum band from Belize.

The value of such music is that it can take one back mentally and emotionally to the foreign site to assist in the analyzing and interpreting of the relevant historical research while you continue to build and travel your bridge between different cultures. Once you have conducted the historical research in the foreign site, you will look at the foreign culture and your own culture through a different lens. Your challenge is to help enable others to look at nursing history through this new lens.

REFERENCES

Bryant, J. (1969). *Health and the developing world.* Ithaca, NY: Cornell University Press.

D'Avanzo, C., & Geissler, E. (2003). *Pocket guide to cultural health assessment.* St. Louis, MO: Mosby.

Masson, V. (1981). *International nursing.* New York: Springer Publishing.

CHAPTER NINE

Working With Primary Sources: An Overview

Keith C. Mages and Julie A. Fairman

> Aug 4th
>
> I am on duty at 7 A.M. With the assistance of one patient served the breakfast. gave after food medicines. washed the bed stands with warm water and ammonia. Took temperatures of all patients in the rear ward. 8 30 gave all of the morning medications. 9 A.M. made poultice for an abscess on an arm. Bathed the same patient with lotion for skin eruption. Gave three fever cases a sponge bath. bathed them thoroughly with alcohol. At 10 A.M. took temperature of typhoid gave medicine. Gave milk to three fever cases. Washed a back with warm water and alcohol. attended to boiling milk and giving it to a patient who is kept on boiled milk alone. because his stomach will not retain any solid food. 11 A.M. gave medications. 11.20 A.M. went to front ward to assist Miss Zimmerman with dressings one could not do alone. Kept there until 11.40 A.M. went to dinner. (Clymer, 1888a, p. 1)

With these morning entries into a small, narrow-ruled notepad, Mary V. Clymer began the documentation of her hospital ward experiences while a student at the Training School for Nurses at the Hospital of the University of Pennsylvania. Her words, penned on August 4, 1888, provide modern historical researchers a vivid glimpse into the past, into the realities of one student nurse's training school life. This chapter aims to introduce the reader to primary sources, to the various resources helpful when looking for primary sources, as well as to the procedural and legal intricacies of conducting historical research with primary sources. Examples are liberally used to assist the reader to gain comfort with, and a more complete understanding of, the nature of historic primary sources.

PRIMARY AND SECONDARY SOURCES DEFINED

Mary Clymer's ward diary is but one manuscript, or handwritten document, housed within the archives of the Barbara Bates Center for the Study of the History of Nursing at the University of Pennsylvania's School of Nursing. As a manuscript, Miss Clymer's diary is considered a primary source. Primary sources are defined as any item having a direct connection with either the creator or user and the time period in which they were crafted or utilized (Presnell, 2007). For many historians, it is the quest for the identification and evaluation of diverse primary sources, combined with the search for relational meaning among such sources, that address pertinent historical questions that really fuels their historical research.

Aside from manuscripts, other primary sources include government documents, hospital records, photographs, newspaper articles, advertisements, census raw data, and even medical instruments. For example, our student nurse Mary Clymer is believed to be the nurse portrayed in Thomas Eakins's painting, *The Agnew Clinic* (Eakins, 1889). In the painting, Miss Clymer stands observantly among a group of physicians undertaking a surgical procedure on a patient within a surgical amphitheater crowded with University of Pennsylvania medical students as Dr. D. Hayes Agnew oversees the entire process. Presented to the University of Pennsylvania Medical School in May of 1889, the same year of Clymer's graduation from the Hospital's Training for Nurses, Eakins's work can be considered another primary source available to those interested in learning more of Mary Clymer (Clymer, 1888b).

Primary sources can be thought of as existing in the following categories: *personal documents, government documents, organizational documents, media communications, artifacts and realia, audio/visual materials,* and *dissertations*. These are not rigid groupings. Some items uncovered may fit into more than one, and alternatively a few primary sources may not seem to fit into any. As such categorization can assist in the conceptualization of primary sources, a brief overview of the primary categories may be helpful (Presnell, 2007, pp. 93–95; Yale University Library, 2007).

Personal documents are usually unique materials created by an individual for record keeping, reflection, or communication. They were not created with a wide audience in mind. Examples of personal documents include journals, letters, and insurance documents. *Government documents* include both public and official government records such as birth and death records, census data, court records, public health records, tax records, legislative hearings, laws, and civil codes (Presnell, 2007). *Organizational documents* record the activities of organizations (businesses, churches, hospitals, etc.) and those individuals who participate in their daily activities. Some examples of organizational documents include church member listings, meeting minutes, and inventory lists. *Media communications* include newspapers, magazines, advertisements, and television news reports. *Artifacts* include any object created by a human being (Soanes & Stevenson, 2005). *Realia* is another term used to describe objects, specifically those used as instructional aids but that were not created with such a purpose in mind (Speake, 1999). Nursing uniforms, thermometers, medication bottles, military and honorary medals, and nursing school pins could all be considered representative of this category. *Audio/visual materials* include original art pieces, photographs, films, posters, maps, blueprints, and recorded speeches. *Dissertations* are original works consisting of an in-depth exploration of a focused topic area that were produced in partial fulfillment of the requirements for doctoral degrees.

Primary sources are not the only type of sources available to those seeking historical information. Secondary sources exist as well. Secondary sources are those items that have used primary sources in their creation (Prytherch, 1995). As such, these sources often offer analyses and interpretations of primary sources (Presnell, 2007). Examples of secondary sources include books, journal articles, and research reports.

Unfortunately, the lines between primary and secondary sources can become blurred at times. Secondary sources that present an intellectual or cultural picture, representative of a particular historic era or point of view are considered primary sources. For example, the textual content of Lavinia Dock and Adelaide Nutting's classic, turn-of-the-20th-century work *A History of Nursing* can be viewed as a secondary source, yet, if the authors' published text (as well as any textual omissions conspicuously left unpublished) are examined to pull forth their underlying attitudes and assumptions, the source becomes a primary one. It is important to discern the difference between primary and secondary sources when undertaking historical research. Generally, primary sources should be the guiding informants regarding your topic of interest with secondary sources used to assist with the identification and comprehension of primary sources. Secondary sources may also be used to help discern the validity and reliability of a primary source; of course the reverse of this is possible as well.

THE HUNT FOR PRIMARY SOURCES

With the wide variety of objects that are considered primary sources, it should not be surprising to learn that primary materials can indeed be found almost anywhere, from family attics and garages to elaborate, state-of-the-art government archival facilities. The majority of collections, those that are known and accessible to the public, exist in three allied institutional spheres: archives, special collection libraries, and museums and historical societies. As each of these institutions have slightly different focuses, the kind of primary source may influence which of these types of collections will prove most useful to the research. As with the categories of primary sources discussed in the previous section, the collections housed within these institutions are not always clearly defined. For instance, a collection identified as a special collection library may indeed be a combination of archive, special collection library, and museum. Indeed, the primary resource can be a sly prey, ever ready to use its environment to confuse the uninitiated hunter.

Archives

Archives are repositories for original manuscripts, records, and documents (Prytherch, 1995). Pearce-Moses (2005) of the Society of American Archivists defines an archive as a collection of

> materials created or received by a person, family, or organization, public or private, in the conduct of their affairs and preserved because of the enduring value contained in the information they contain or as evidence of the functions and responsibilities of their creator.

Archives may exist as a stand-alone entity, or they may be affiliated with a national or local government, university, business, or hospital. The National Historical Publications and Research Commission's *Directory of Archives and Manuscript Repositories in the United States,* 2nd ed., provides a good overview of over 4,500 archival collections across the United States, but, as this printed resource has not been updated since the 1988, its data may be a bit dated (Mann, 1998).

On the Internet, the *Repositories of Primary Sources* (http://www.uidaho.edu/special-collections/Other.Repositories.html) provides a current, frequently updated, database of archival and manuscript collections around the world, with an especially comprehensive overview of collections in the United States (Figure 9.1; Abraham, 2007). Providing hyperlinks to the Web page of each respective collection, this resource presents a useful way to browse the holdings of institutions of interest.

Repositories of Primary Sources

A listing of over 5000 websites describing holdings of manuscripts, archives, rare books historical photographs, and other primary sources for the research scholar. All links have been tested for correctness and appropriateness.
Links added or revised within the last thirty days or so are marked *{New}*. Please use this form or e-mail to add entries, provide corrections, or make comments on its utility. Those who have recently submitted new and revised entries are acknowledged. Guidelines for the inclusion of sites on this list are available.
Compiled by Terry Abraham.

- Western United States and Canada
- Eastern United States and Canada: States and Provinces A-M
- Eastern United States and Canada: States and Provinces N-Z
- Latin America and the Caribbean
- Europe A-M
- Europe N-Z
- Asia and the Pacific
- Africa and the Near East
- Additional Lists
- State, Province, Country Index
- Integrated Index/List.

January 2007/Other.Repositories.html/Since1995 /0625257

© Copyright 1995-2007 Terry Abraham

FIGURE 9.1 Screenshot of the Repositories of Primary Sources homepage. Used with permission of Terry Abraham.

When looking for archival primary sources regarding a specific person or topic, various online resources are available. The National Union Catalog of Manuscript Collections, a gateway to the RLG Union Catalog provided by the Library of Congress (2005) (http://www.loc.gov/coll/nucmc/rlinsearch.html), provides a cost-free Web-mediated method of searching for archival collections. WorldCat (http://www.worldcat.org) provides an additional portal for searching the RLG Union Catalog. WorldCat also provides the researcher with the opportunity to search the catalog holdings of over 10,000 libraries and archives worldwide (OCLC Online Computer Library Center, Inc., 2007a).

ArchiveGrid offers an alternative to the aforementioned portals that search the RLG Union Catalog (Figure 9.2; OCLC Online Computer Library Center, Inc., 2007b). This subscription-based resource features descriptions of nearly 1 million historical documents, with the collection summaries, notes, and contact information clearly presented. Researchers should check with their institution to see if their academic library subscribes to ArchiveGrid.

Special Collection Libraries

Special collection libraries work to acquire unique and rare textual materials for scholarly research. Many of these libraries specialize in the collection and preservation of antiquarian books and journals in specific

Lecture Notes, c. 1886-1889.

Clymer, Mary U.
Lecture Notes, c. 1886-1889.
.2 linear ft.

Contact an archivist to learn more about access to materials in this collection

University of Pennsylvania - Center for the Study of the History of Nursing
Location: Center for the study of the history of Nursing, School of Nursing, University of Pennsylvania, 307 Nursing Education Building, Philadelphia, PA 19104-6096
Location: PU-N
Call Number: MC 16

Notes and Summaries:

Nursing student at the Hospital of the University of Pennsylvania. Clymer is the nurse featured in the Thomas Eakins's portrait of the Agnew Clinic at the University of Pennsylvania's School of Medicine.

This collection consists of Mary U. Clymers's lecture notes as a nursing student at the Hospital of the University of Pennsylvania. Part of one volume describes Clymers's ward duties and portrays daily activities of the 19th century hospital ward.

Unpublished finding aid in repository.

Preferred Citation: Mary U. Clymer Lecture Notes, Center for the Study of the History of Nursing, School of Nursing, University of Pennsylvania.

This collection covers:

University of Pennsylvania. Hospital School of Nursing.

FIGURE 9.2 Screenshot of the ArchiveGrid entry regarding lecture notes penned by Mary Clymer. Courtesy of ArchiveGrid.

subject areas such as history of medicine or Shakespearean works. Special collection libraries may exist independently, as part of a larger library, or within a university. Once again, WorldCat is an excellent database to turn to when looking for applicable primary sources. Many special collection libraries have made the catalogs of their holdings available via WorldCat. Another resource, one with great relevance for historical health sciences research, is the *Directory of History of Medicine Collections* (http://www.nlm.nih.gov/hmd/directory/directoryhome.html). This database, created by the National Library of Medicine, History of Medicine Division (2006), lists the contact information, Internet address, and overview of the holdings of many U.S. health sciences special library collections.

Museums and Historical Societies

Museums and historical societies are another source of primary materials. Museums are an especially rich source for artifacts and realia. A good place to search for museums, of any focus, is the American Association of

Museums (2007) Web page (http://www.aam-us.org/museumresources/accred/list.cfm). When looking for medical and health science museums, the Dittrick Medical History Center's (2006) Web site provides an excellent starting point (http://www.case.edu/artsci/dittrick/site2/links/).

Historical societies offer primary resources of local interest, with an eye on the preservation and dissemination of local history and genealogic resources. Unfortunately, no master Web site exists to aid in the search for local historical societies. If interested in learning more of the resources housed within local historical societies, try a quick Internet search using a favorite search engine, or alternatively take a chance with the phone book.

MAKING USE OF PRIMARY SOURCES

When a researcher identifies a collection of interest, they should take a few moments to contact the institution housing the documents. A short inquiry to verify hours of reading room/museum operation, reference procedures, and the suitability of the identified primary source to your area of interest saves a great deal of time and frustration. Smaller collections may have limited staffing and reference hours, so a reference appointment may need to be made. Also, feel free to discuss the research topic with the archivist, librarian, or curator during the initial contact. These individuals are experts at finding information within their respective collections and can indeed be excellent resources when looking for additional information. One should always be as specific as possible when describing the research to be conducted—the clearer the request, the more fulfilling the results!

Remember, many items housed in archives, special collection libraries, and museums are noncirculating; researchers should bring a pencil and pad or laptop with them (if the site allows such devices) and be sure to leave plenty of time to read the documents and explore the collection finding aid. Finding aids contain several informative components that can enhance navigation through the collections. Good finding aids will identify the size of the collection (number of boxes or linear feet), its provenance (or history before coming to the archive), any access restrictions (some sensitive material may not be available for research until a future date), citation, biographical sketch of the author, along with a summary of the collection's contents.

Upon arrival at a repository, expect to follow certain institutional specific protocols before gaining access to any documents. At the Barbara Bates Center, researchers are asked to complete an "Application to Use Center Holdings," a form used to compile statistical and research topic summaries that ask for pertinent identifying and research information (Figure 9.3).

Barbara Bates Center for The Study of The History of Nursing

School of Nursing, University of Pennsylvania, 307 NEB, Philadelphia, PA 19104-6096

APPLICATION TO USE CENTER HOLDINGS

Name (printed)

Local address

Local Telephone

Permanent Address:

Telephone:
e-mail address:
FAX number:
Profession/Occupation

Please check one:
( ) UP Undergraduate
( ) UP Graduate Student
( ) UP Faculty/Staff
( ) Non-UP Undergraduate
( ) Non-UP Graduate Student
( ) Non-UP Faculty/Staff
( ) Nursing alumni association member
( ) Publisher
( ) Genealogist
( ) Other:

Institutional/Organizational Affiliation:

If candidate for degree, give degree sought:

Please describe the purpose of your research:

Please identify collections of specific interest:

Validation of identification (driver's license, student or faculty i.d., etc.)—Required for research room users:

Data from this form will be used to compile statistical and research topic summaries. We attempt to inform researchers working in related fields of similar research interest. Can we mention your name and information about your research topic to other interested scholars? Yes _____ No _____

Barbara Bates Center for The Study of The History of Nursing (*continued*)

I agree to indemnify and hold harmless The Trustees of the University of Pennsylvania, its officers, trustees, employees and agents from and against all claims, actions, damages and costs, including attorney's fees, arising out of my use of the materials in the Center.

I have received a copy of the Center's rules, which I have read, I understand, and agree to abide by in the use of the Center's materials.

Signature Date

Approved by:

FIGURE 9.3 Duplication of the Barbara Bates Center for the Study of the History of Nursing form "Application to Use Center Holdings." Used with permission of the BBCSHN.

Additionally, before utilizing any of the Center's resources, researchers are asked to read the "Rules Governing the Use of Center Materials" (Figure 9.4). This form outlines the items that may be brought into the reading room with the researcher (materials necessary for research, e.g., a pencil, tablet, laptop, hand scanner, and usually not a book bag or any other tote bag or handbag), along with the Center's registration, publication, and photoduplication protocols.

Once situated within the reading room, if at an archive and have not done so already, take a moment to read over the finding aid for the collection of interest. Next, begin to carefully read through the primary resource. At times, an archives or special collection library may provide a photocopied version of the original document or book. This is usually done for the preservation of either extremely fragile or popular materials to reduce the handling of the originals. As a researcher reads through the documents, they typically think about the following question: How does the information contained within this document contribute to the research? If the document indeed provides information relevant to the historical questions framing the research project, continue studying the documents and consider the following (DoHistory.org, 2000): *What is it (diary, personal letter, patient record, etc.)? Who created it? Who was the intended audience? For what purpose was it created? When was it created? Where was it created? How was it created? Is there anything we do not know about this document?*

Barbara Bates Center for The Study of The History of Nursing

University of Pennsylvania – School of Nursing – Nursing Education Building – Philadelphia, PA 19104-6096 – (215) 898-4502

RULES GOVERNING THE USE OF CENTER MATERIALS

Introduction

The materials housed in the Barbara Bates Center for the Study of the History of Nursing are noncirculating. Some of them are in fragile condition and largely irreplaceable. Therefore, certain precautions are necessary. The following rules are designed to instruct readers in the special handling procedures needed to preserve these materials for future scholars.

Materials Brought to the Reading Room

The researcher may bring only those materials needed for research and a pencil to the reading room tables. All coats, briefcases, and other items should be checked with the administrative assistant in the reading room.

Permission to Examine

Permission to examine manuscript material will be granted to qualified researchers upon completion of the application form and agreeing to abide by the rules governing the use of manuscripts. Such permissions are granted subject to whatever restrictions may have been placed on the material by the donors, depositors, or the repository. Case anonymity must be respected regarding student files, employment files, and any other files relating to personal matters.

Registration

Researchers must fill out and sign an application form once each fiscal year (July 1–June 30), and must provide acceptable identification (driver's license or i.d. card with photograph). The Daily Register must be signed each visit by all researchers.

Protection of Materials

A researcher is responsible for the safeguarding of any materials made available to him/her in the reading room. Researchers may

Barbara Bates Center for The Study of The History of Nursing (*continued*)

not remove materials from the reading room for any purpose or rearrange the order in which they are delivered. The use of any kind of pen is prohibited. Manuscripts may not be leaned on, written on, folded, or handled in any way likely to damage them. In certain cases, researchers may be required to use microfilm or photocopies of manuscripts when such copies are available. Eating and smoking are prohibited in the reading room. Researchers are requested to wash their hands before using materials and avoid using any creams or lotions thereafter as grease can transfer to the materials causing considerable damage. Researchers will be asked to wear cotton gloves when handling photographic holdings and other items in which conditions merit the use of gloves.

Permission to Publish

Permission to examine materials is not an authorization to publish them. Separate written application for permission to publish must be made to the Center. Researchers who plan eventual publication of their work should inquire concerning general restrictions on publication before beginning their research. To the extent that it may properly do so, the Center will ordinarily grant the usual publication rights to applicants. In granting permission to publish, the Center does not surrender its own right after that to publish any of the materials from its collection or grant permission to others to publish them. If the Center grants permission to publish, the location of the cited material shall be indicated in the published work. A free copy of all publications that rely heavily on the collections in the Center should be presented to the Center upon publication. The Center does not assume any responsibility for infringement of copyright in the materials held by others.

Recommended Citation

For citations in published or unpublished papers, this repository should be listed as the Center for the Study of the History of Nursing, School of Nursing, University of Pennsylvania. Manuscript collections should be cited as in the following example: "Visiting Nurse Society of Philadelphia Records, Barbara Bates Center for the Study of the History of Nursing, School of Nursing, University of Pennsylvania."

Barbara Bates Center for The Study of The History of Nursing (*continued*)

Photoduplication

The Center will consider requests for the photoduplication of material when such duplication can be done without injury to the material, and does not violate copyright or donor restrictions. Single copies will be provided for the researcher's personal reference use. The photocopy/photograph must not be further reproduced. Supplying a photocopy/photograph is not an authorization to publish.

Exclusive Rights

Exclusive rights to examine or publish will not be granted.

FIGURE 9.4 Duplication of the Barbara Bates Center for the Study of the History of Nursing form "Rules Governing the Use of Center Materials." Used with permission of the BBCSHN.

For example, when examining Mary Clymer's ward diary, the following information can be gathered (Clymer, 1888a):

1. *What is it (diary, personal letter, patient record, etc.)?* Ward diary drafted by Mary Clymer as a student nurse at the Training School for Nurses at the Hospital of the University of Pennsylvania.
2. *Who created it?* Mary V. Clymer. Sometimes incorrectly identified as Mary U. Clymer (Clymer, 1888b).
3. *Who was the intended audience?* The ward supervisor.
4. *For what purpose was it created?* To document Mary Clymer's clinical activities as a student while on the hospital ward, including her assigned duties, the care she provided, and her interactions with staff nurses and other hospital employees. It is assumed to have served as a way for the ward supervisor to evaluate Clymer's work.
5. *When was it created?* August 4–November 19, 1888.
6. *Where was it created?* Hospital of the University of Pennsylvania, Philadelphia, PA.
7. *How was it created?* Handwritten in pencil.
8. *Is there anything we do not know about this document?* Why does the collection only have one of Miss Clymer's ward notebooks, covering just 3 1/2 months of 1888? As she was a student up until her graduation in the spring of 1889, did she write any others? Are they perhaps in another archive? With a family member still?

In general, many researchers develop their own note system to keep the information obtained from each of their sources in some sort of manageable format. Always keep accurate notes regarding where particular data fragments were obtained (e.g., an archival document's file number or box number, an antiquarian book's call number). Questions regarding a primary source could surface at anytime, including issues pertaining to the validity and reliability of these documents. The following questions may help to address these issues (DoHistory.org, 2000): *Does this source raise any questions? Does this document reference similar sources that could provide further relevant information? Does the information within this document seem to support or refute previously gathered information?*

PRIMARY SOURCES AND LEGAL SOURCES AND LEGAL ISSUES: MARY CLYMER AND HIPAA

The excerpt from the Clymer diary in the beginning of the chapter contains information about the care of patients. At the top of the entry is the date, and a specific time is noted shortly thereafter. There is talk of fever cases, a patient with a boil, and of a "Miss Zimmerman," a student nurse or perhaps a graduate nurse who needed help redressing patient wounds. Most of this information is nonspecific, and there are no identifiers that a researcher could use to find a specific patient.

Before 2003, a historian requesting access to a source such as the Clymer diary might be armed with their specific research questions and little else. They only needed to make an appointment with the research center administrator, read the diary, and then analyze the respective content and integrate the data into their writings. After April 2003, when the Health Insurance Portability and Accountability Act (HIPAA) of 1996 (P. L. 104–191) formally went into effect, researchers were required to consider several new and different steps before they gained access to collections.

Congress first passed HIPAA in 1996 to make it easier for American employees to change jobs without losing eligibility for health benefits at the new job based on pre-existing health condition exclusions in their benefits contracts. The Act was also meant to reduce fraud and health care costs by "facilitating the electronic exchange of data related to financial and administrative transactions," such as payments from Medicare and Medicaid (Lawrence, 2007, p. 5; Novak, 2003; U.S. Department of Health and Human Services, 2003). The part of HIPAA that is most important to the work of historians is the Privacy Rule, which sets up standards for protecting individually identifiable health information (IIHI) and definitions of important terminology (U.S. Department of Health and Human Services, 2007). HIPAA "has no sense of the past" and is retroactive, covering all existing records and their data no matter how old, on both dead and living subjects, and has no guidelines for how long records of the deceased must be protected (Ericson & Koste, 2003; National Committee on Vital and Health Statistics, 2005; U.S. Department of Health and Human Services, 2003). It is an attempt to apply 21st-century guidelines to historical documents that were written in a complex and distant past.

The first question for researchers to consider when they locate a repository that might have records to help answer important historical questions is the following: *Is this archive a covered entity?* According to HIPAA, a covered entity is a "health plan, a health care information clearinghouse, or a health care provider [and or their business agents] who transmits information in electronic form in connection with a transaction (typically billing or payment transactions) for which the Department of Health and Human Services (HHS) has adopted a standard" (U.S. Department of Health and Human Services, 2003, p. 3). If the archive resides in a covered entity, it itself is a covered entity. Currently, operating hospitals and dental and physician offices that submit patient information in electronic form for billing and other purposes to HHS are considered covered entities. Old hospital or physician records, even though they do not exist in electronic form, are considered held in a covered entity if they were stored in hospital storage or a hospital archive. If they were transferred to an archive before 2003, for example, to the National Library of Medicine, which is an uncovered entity, the old records are "uncovered." Most universities are considered hybrid entities, that is, with both covered and uncovered entities because they can separate out health care activities from those that are not (Lawrence, 2007).

If the archive is not a covered entity, as the one holding the Clymer diary, then the HIPAA Privacy Rule does not come into play. If it *is* a covered entity, then the next question is: *Do the records requested by the researcher contain Protected Health Information (PHI)?* This information is a subset of "individually identifiable health information transmitted by electronic media, maintained in electronic media, or transmitted or maintained in any other form or medium" (U.S. Department of Health and Human Services, n.d., p. 2). PHI includes "demographic or other data relating to the past, present, and future physical or mental health condition of a patient, or the provision of care or payment to a health provider, health plan, employer or health clearinghouse," created by a health provider, health plan, employer or health clearinghouse (U.S. Department of Health and Human Services., n.d., p. 8). This includes photographs of people that are readily identified as patients and those of doctors and nurses with patients. The HIPAA Privacy Rule only applies to information (rather than records) "that is the responsibility of the covered entity *and* its IIHI" (Lawrence, 2007, p. 12).

If the Clymer diary were the responsibility of a covered entity, would the opening passage be considered to be containing PHI? First, the diary was created by a care provider—a nursing student. It also contains information on services, although not on payments: "gave milk to three fever patients...attended to boiling milk and giving it to patient...because his stomach will not retain any solid food...." But, does this excerpt (which is recognizably not the whole of which this determination would be made) include unique identifiers? There are 18 unique elements enumerated by the Privacy Rule that could identify a patient, relative, employee, or household member, including names, geographic areas smaller than a state, birth date, all ages over 89 years, full-face photographic images, and addresses. The Clymer entry includes a date, but it is specific only to her work and not to the admission of a patient. There are no names, birthdates, or addresses of Clymer or the patients. There are no specific identifiers in the excerpt that could individually identify the patients Clymer cared for on that date. There were probably numerous fever, typhoid, or stomach patients, and although these patients were in an area as specific as a hospital ward, the narrative does not specify which one. And many hospital wards had "back rooms." If the diary included information that provided details, for example, "Mr. Jones in Ward H was admitted on August 3rd after he was found inebriated and lying in a ditch by his home on 217 Front Street," then this diary would be said to include PHI.

If the diary was the responsibility of a covered entity, then several options would be available to the researcher in order to access the documents. To begin with, we know Miss Clymer is no longer alive, as she completed her nurse training probably in 1889. Neither are the patients. According to the Privacy Rule, the records of living and deceased persons are treated differently, and there are certain conditions for accessing the records of deceased persons, as the Privacy Rule extends perpetual protection. To obtain access to the records of a deceased subject, the researcher must first disclose either orally or in writing to the entity that the use or disclosure sought is solely for research purposes and only for the PHI of the descendants. The individual's death must then be documented at the request of the covered entity (which some have suggested means it is up to the covered entity to decide how this is done), especially if the subject was less than 100 years old. Finally, the researcher must assure the entity that the protected information is necessary for the research project. Typical access policies are not that different (Novak, 2003).

A researcher who wants to examine the Clymer diary (depending on the particular covered entity) might have to present a copy of a proposal, particular research questions, or an updated curricula vita to document their interest and agree, again either orally or in writing, not to study Miss Clymer's descendants or those of any patient with IIHI. If a covered entity decides to give historians access to nonredacted documents (e.g., the PHI is not taken out or is disclosed), the covered entity must have assurances from the researcher that they will do their own redacting when the subject's identity is not necessary to the research, e.g., not using patient names, or by creating pseudonyms or codes. They must also promise to take responsibility for keeping the information confidential. In other words, the researcher must agree not to disclose the identity to others. In some places, access to these types of documents and their use depends on the covered entities "trust or distrust" of historical inquiry (Lawrence, 2007, p. 24). In other places, the entity may demand the researcher destroy notes containing PHI after the project is finished and that the entity itself has the right to review manuscripts to ensure there is no possible identification of individuals (U.S. Department of Health and Human Services, 2004).

If the Clymer diary was written in the 1950s and Miss Clymer and presumably the patients were still alive, there are several ways a researcher can gain access to records containing PHI, although this is a more complicated process. And, some archives, even those uncovered, are applying access terms to the records of the deceased that are similar to those for documents of those who are still alive. If the Clymer diary contained PHI and the archival staff already de-identified all 18 elements defining PHI, perhaps for a previous researcher, then access is allowed. De-identifying a document requires an incredible amount of labor. First, the archival staff must examine the documents and then de-identify the information by making a copy and removing (e.g., through blackout) the PHI. Sometimes this is not possible because the documents requested may be too fragile to copy. For more recent records, typically post-HIPAA, individuals may authorize a covered entity to disclose or use their PHI for specific research purposes (this is not the same as informed consent; Lusk & Sacharski, 2005). Clymer's diary obviously doesn't fit into that category, but if it did, authorization would only be for permission to use the records with PHI for a very defined project at a particular time for a particular historical question.

Another way for researchers to gain access to records containing PHI is to apply for a HIPAA waiver from an Institutional Review Board (IRB) or a Privacy Board (Privacy Boards were intended to take some of the work pressure off Institutional Review Boards and consist of at least two members who have no financial interest in the project they are asked to examine.) (Lawrence, 2007). As any IRB or Privacy Board will suffice, the researcher should probably submit their proposals to their home IRBs first, which will determine if the proposal addresses the HIPAA privacy requirements and if an HIPAA waiver is allowed. But, many covered entities may require a resubmission to their own IRBs or Privacy Boards, depending on the advice from their legal representatives (Health Privacy Project, 2002).

To issue a waiver, the entity through the IRB or designated board or officer must ascertain that the disclosure of the information renders minimal or no privacy risk to the individual of the record. There are several criteria that must be met in order for a waiver to be granted. These include plans to protect identifiers from improper use and disclosure, a plan to destroy the identifiers when the project is completed, and written assurances that the PHI will not be disclosed to any other entity unless required for authorized oversight. There must also be some justification that the research could not practically be conducted without the waiver and access to and use of the PHI (Health Privacy Project, 2002). At some repositories such as the National Library of Medicine (a noncovered entity but one that has developed policies that address HIPAA issues), policies granting access for even the records of the deceased require researchers to "agree in writing to maintain the confidentiality of the information and to adhere to the conditions of access imposed" by the library (U.S. Department of Health and Human Services, 2004).

Following these stipulations should not be that onerous for historians, as the expectations are "largely commonsense preparations" (Lawrence, 2007, p. 26). For example, keeping the Clymer notes in a locked drawer or file cabinet, or on the drive of a password protected laptop should probably be part of the researcher's basic method anyway. And, although a researcher could use Clymer's name in a presentation (as the Bates Center is not a covered entity, and her portrait in the Eakins painting is part of the public domain), in cases where the subject was younger and part of a covered entity, pseudonyms would suffice.

As long as historians understand the regulations, even in a very basic sense, they should be able to access documents to continue their research. The HIPAA was not intended to make life difficult for historians, but because of the complexity of the legal language and the vagueness of the various subsections, the result has been an individualized response as each archive and repository tries to understand what the HIPAA means for them and the researchers who use their collections. There have been indirect consequences as each archive attempts to define their status and their response to the collections. The regulations have been particularly damaging to researchers interested in the history of children in some form (Hinderer, 2004).

The regulations, despite the protests of many historians, are here to stay, and although some amendments to them may occur over time, they in fact offer an opportunity to standardize access to historical documents and protect the privacy of individuals. Additionally, HIPAA is too narrow to affect most historians because the vast majority of libraries and repositories do not sit in covered entities. A researcher must appropriately use historical documents and pay attention to personal information contained in letters and diaries that were not intended for public reading. This approach helps maintain a sometimes delicate balance of access to records containing PHI with the need to protect a subject's privacy. Historians would do well to respond to this tension no matter where the materials reside.

Ultimately, the hard part of historical research is not tracking primary sources, nor is it using them legally within the confines of HIPAA; the difficult part is finding those sources that help answer specific historical questions. As historians examine primary documents, they are trying to learn as much as possible about their topic of research. Primary sources provide the closest links to the lives of our predecessors; it is essential that anyone who hopes to inform and enhance their understanding of a particular historical subject be well versed in the various aspects of these vital resources.

REFERENCES

Abraham T. (2007). *Repository of primary sources.* Retrieved June 12, 2007, from http://www.uidaho.edu/special-collections/Other.Repositories.html

American Association of Museums. (2007). *List of accredited museums.* Retrieved June 13, 2007, from http://www.aam-us.org/museumresources/accred/list.cfm

Clymer, M. V. (1888a). Ward notebook. *Mary V. Clymer papers.* Philadelphia: University of Pennsylvania, School of Nursing, Barbara Bates Center for the Study of the History of Nursing.

Clymer, M. V. (1888b). Finding aid. *Mary V. Clymer papers.* Philadelphia: University of Pennsylvania, School of Nursing, Barbara Bates Center for the Study of the History of Nursing.

Dittrick Medical History Center. (2006). *Medical museums, archives, and libraries in the United States.* Retrieved June 13, 2007, from http://www.case.edu/artsci/dittrick/site2/links/

DoHistory.org. (2000). Using primary sources. *DoHistory (History Toolkit).* Retrieved June 13, 2007, from http://dohistory.org/on_your_own/toolkit/primarySources.html

Eakins, T. (1889). *The Agnew Clinic.* Oil on canvas. Philadelphia: University of Pennsylvania.

Ericson, T., & Koste, J. (2003, October 22). Letter sent on behalf of the Society of American Archivists to Health and Human Services Secretary, Tommy Thompson. *The Watermark: Newsletter of the Archivist and Librarians in the History of the Health Sciences, XXVII* (1). Retrieved June 10, 2007, from http://www.library.ucla.edu/biomed/alhhs/

Health Privacy Project, Institute for Health Research and Policy, Georgetown University. (2002, September 13). *Summary of HIPAA Privacy Rule.* Retrieved June 1, 2007, from http://www.healthprivacy.org/usr_doc/RegSummary2002.pdf

Hinderer M. (2004). Historians, privacy, and archives. *Newsletter of the Society for the History of Children and Youth, 3*(winter). Retrieved May 27, 2007, from http://www.h-net.org/~child/newsletters/newsletter3/privacy.html

Lawrence, S. C. (2007). Access anxiety: HIPAA and historical research. *Journal of the History of Medicine and Allied Science.* Advance access published online on January 4, 2007. Retrieved June 7, 2007, from http://jhmas.oxfordjournals.org/cgi/reprint/jrl048v1

The Library of Congress. (2005). *National Union Catalog of Manuscript Collections.* Retrieved June 12, 2007, from http://www.loc.gov/coll/nucmc/rlinsearch.html

Lusk, B., & Sacharski, S. (2005). Dead or alive: HIPAA's impact on nursing historical research. *Nursing History Review, 13,* 189–197.

Mann, T. (1998). *The Oxford guide to library research.* New York: Oxford University Press, 261.

National Committee on Vital and Health Statistics, Subcommittee on Privacy and Confidentiality, Panel 3-Decendent Health Information. (January 11, 2005). *The impact on the HIPPA Privacy Rule on the ability to access and utilize archives. Testimony of Nancy McCall, The Johns Hopkins Medical Institutions.* Retrieved June 1, 2007, from http://www.ncvhs.hhs.gov/050111p6.pdf

National Library of Medicine, History of Medicine Division. (2006). *Directory of History of Medicine Collections.* Retrieved June 13, 2007, from http://www.nlm.nih.gov/hmd/directory/directoryhome.html

Novak, S. E. (2003). The Health Insurance Portability and Accountability Act of 1996: Its implications for history of medicine collections. *The Watermark: Newsletter of the Archivist and Librarians in the History of the Health Sciences, XXVI* (3). Retrieved June 10, 2007, from http://www.library.ucla.edu/biomed/alhhs/articlehealthinsuranceportability.html

OCLC Online Computer Library Center, Inc. (2007a). *WorldCat.* Retrieved June 19, 2007, from http://www.worldcat.org

OCLC Online Computer Library Center, Inc. (2007b). *ArchiveGrid.* Retrieved June 12, 2007, from http://www.archivegrid.org

Pearce-Moses, R. (2005). Archives. *A glossary of archival and records terminology* (Society of American Archivists). Retrieved May 29, 2007, from http://www.archivists.org/glossary/term_details.asp?DefinitionKey=156

Presnell, J. L. (2007). *The information-literate historian: A guide to research for history students.* New York: Oxford University Press.

Prytherch, R. (1995). *Harrod's librarians' dictionary.* Brookfield, VT: Ashgate Publishing Co.

Soanes, C., & Stevenson A. (Eds.). (2005). *The Oxford dictionary of English.* New York: Oxford University Press.

Speake, J. (Ed). (1999). *The Oxford essential dictionary of foreign terms in English.* New York: Berkley Books.

U.S. Department of Health and Human Services. (n.d.). *Protecting personal health information in research: Understanding the HIPAA privacy rules.* Retrieved May 26, 2007, from http://www.research.usf.edu/cs/hipaa_forms/nihguide.pdf

U.S. Department of Health and Human Services. (2003). *Summary of the HIPAA Privacy Rule.* Retrieved June 10, 2007, from http://www.hhs.gov/ocr/privacysummary.pdf

U.S. Department of Health and Human Services. (2007). *What does the HIPAA Privacy Act do?* Retrieved May 1, 2007, from http://www.hhs.gov/hipaafaq/about/187.html

U.S. Department of Health and Human Services, Public Health Services, National Library of Medicine, History of Medicine Division. (2004). *Access to Health Information of Individuals.* Retrieved June 1, 2007, from http://www.nlm.nih.gov/hmd/manuscripts/phi.pdf

Yale University Library. (2007). The formats of primary sources. *Primary sources at Yale.* Retrieved June 10, 2007, from http://www.library.yale.edu/in struction/primsource.html

CHAPTER TEN

"The Truth About the Past?" The Art of Working With Archival Materials

Christine Hallett

The core work of the historian is the interpretation of textual data. Although modern approaches to the collection of historical sources, such as the life history interview, are becoming increasingly important, most historians still spend much of their time "searching the archives" (Kirby, 1997). But what does the concept of the *search* really mean? Clearly, archive work involves more than simply collecting material to be later somehow "used" as a piece of history. How does the historian decide what to search for, what to retain, and what to discard? Once the source materials—the bedrock of the historian's work—have been collected, how are decisions made about what material to include in the history that is written, and how to order it?

The central element of any good piece of historical writing is a scholarly argument. A book or article that simply recounts supposed facts or events from the past can be seen as chronicle, not history. At the other end of the spectrum, a piece of imaginative writing that incorporates a few historically accurate details can probably be considered a piece of creative writing. Historians make certain claims for their work that set them apart from chroniclers and creative writers. Among these is the claim that a piece of historical work offers some insight into the past (and in doing so provides perspective on the present Maggs, 1987; Rafferty, 1991). And embedded within this claim is the notion that history writing conveys the *truth* about the past; a notion that some consider naïve, but others see as essential (Davies, 1980, 1995; Lusk, 1997; Rafferty, 1997).

This chapter considers whether it is possible for historians to use the material available in archives to write history that approaches the *truth* about the past. It addresses the question of whether it is the historian's goal to come to grips with a single unassailable truth, or whether there are always multiple truths, represented by a range of historical interpretations. It considers, furthermore, if truth does indeed exist, whether it is more likely to be found in the intentions of those individuals who produced the historical sources or in the interpretations that are placed on them by historians.

The chapter will focus on the dilemmas that face historians when approaching any piece of work. A historical study normally begins with a question, or set of questions, to be answered—or at least with a broad area to be explored. The first decision the historian must make relates to nature of the sources themselves. The researcher must appreciate the perspectives of those who created them and the apparent intentions behind their production (Firby, 1993; Fitzpatrick, 2001). They must be aware of their own interpretive approach to these texts (Hallett, 1997; Marwick, 2001; Rafferty, 1991). A number of approaches are possible, and these range from the most straightforward—the empirical—to the most complex—the postmodern. This hierarchy of complexity is, however, in itself, rather misleading. A piece of ostensibly *empirical* history, which privileges *facts* over interpretation and may claim to be free of prejudice or bias, may often contain a hidden ideology, which may sometimes not be apparent even to the author (Jenkins, 1991). Similarly, a *relativist* piece, in which the author openly acknowledges their ideological or theoretical perspective, may focus so deliberately on its own standpoint that it fails to do full justice to the intentions of those who produced the source materials it uses (Carr, 1961; Collingwood, 1994; Marwick, 2001).

THE SEARCH FOR RELEVANT SOURCE MATERIALS

A historical study usually begins with an idea or question, which then leads a researcher to a relevant body of source materials. The origins of historical research questions are often mysterious. Often, the question that underpins a piece of historical work will have emerged from a close reading of the secondary sources—those historical works that have been produced by other practicing researchers. Other questions may have very personal origins—they will have emerged out of the life-experiences of the researcher and then been applied to, and compared with, the secondary literature. Most historians will have formed their research questions from a range of sources—personal and academic. Many are largely unaware of what their questions are and see their work as an essentially exploratory enterprise, out of which questions will emerge and then be answered. Most, however, will have unspoken, half-formed questions in their minds (Gaddis, 2002; Hamilton, 1993; Lowenthal, 1985).

One of the ways to ensure that a historical project is rigorous and worthwhile is to be clear about what questions are underpinning it. These can be flexible and may change as the archives begin to be unearthed, perhaps producing surprises that shift the whole focus of a body of work. Yet, working consciously is vital. Being clear about what one's questions are, yet, being prepared to shift and remodel these in the light of the emerging source materials safeguards rigor in historical work.

Keith Jenkins referred to historical sources as "traces of the past"; these are not evidence and do not become evidence until they have been used in some way to support an argument (Jenkins, 1991, 1995). They are not "the past"; they merely offer us some clues as to what the past may have been like. What traces we choose to view is dictated by both chance and choice. Some sources may have been accidentally destroyed, or may simply have decayed. More often, though, the survival of source materials depends on conscious decisions by human beings. People—whether acting as members of official organizations, or as private individuals—decide what to preserve and what to discard (McGann, 1997). Those documents that are preserved may ultimately be sent to a public archive, where a further decision will be taken about how much to retain. Some archives only have space for a sample of records, rather than for a whole collection. Similarly, national libraries may not be able to retain copies of every publication that comes to their attention (Marwick, 1989, 2001).

USING OFFICIAL ARCHIVES

Modern archives in developed countries are remarkably easy to use. The British National Archives is typical of an official archive that provides a range of online services for the public. The use of these services can make it easier for the researcher to prepare for their visit. The archive provides a complete online catalog. It is possible to undertake a partial online registration, however, it must be completed in person at the archive. Once registered, it is possible to use a reader's ticket to access saved searches and to make advance orders. As with many official archives, the British National Archives is a valuable repository of sources that are useful for studying the history of national organizations, for pursuing family history, or for tracing records relating to individuals. It contains British census records and information about births, marriages, and deaths. For anyone studying the history of nursing, the British National Archives holds important records relating to nurse registration, along with material on individual nurses and on hospitals and training schools. It also contains particularly detailed records of the armed forces, and therefore is useful for the study of army nursing (http://www.nationalarchives.gov.uk).

The National Archives of Australia has a "RecordSearch" facility, which, its Web site states, "contains descriptions of over 6 million records, created by 9000 Australian Government agencies." Like the British National Archives, it is possible to "search...as a guest," or to register "as an archives user." This archive provides a particularly clear description on its Web site of the scope of a national archive:

> Spanning almost 200 years, the collection is a vast and rich resource for the study of Australian history, society and people, most records in the collection are files. But there are also significant holdings of photographs, posters maps, architectural drawings, films, playscripts, musical scores and sound recordings...Each year thousands of people use the collection to do research. They include academics, genealogists, local historians, hobbyists, journalists, students, professional historians and lawyers. Whatever the purpose of your research or the nature of your enquiry, the Archives welcomes your interest in the collection. (Australian Government National Archives of Australia, n.d.)

On another page, the Web site explains that its purpose is "holding on to our history." It is emphasized that the high standard of record keeping helps "government to account to the public ensuring that evidence is available to support people's rights and entitlements and that future generations will have a meaningful record of the past."

This record-keeping element of the archivist's work is of central importance. It is important to be aware, as a historian, that archivists have a dual role that can create some tension for them. They are the preservers of a range of traces of the past. But they also make these traces accessible. *Preservation* can often conflict with *access,* and this can create frustrating experiences for historical researchers, particularly when time is short. Sometimes, archivists may refuse to photocopy, or reproduce in other ways, material that can seem vital to a project. In these cases, there is no alternative but to spend time in the archive itself. For this reason, archive work can become an expensive and time-consuming pursuit, and it is difficult to pursue some projects without funding.

Most official archives are currently engaged in digitization projects, which make available accurate photographic representations of some of their sources. The Web site of the Australian National Archives permits users to make requests for digitization, but this and other archives will normally only digitize what are viewed as large collections of records that have clear national significance. The Royal College of Nursing Archives of the United Kingdom has digitized the complete run of the *British Journal of Nursing,* providing valuable online access to the journal (http://www.rcn.org.uk). Similarly, The National Library and Archives of Canada recently completed a digitization project of First World War nurses titled "Canada's Nursing Sisters," which provides online access to the letters and diaries of six nurses who served with the Canadian Army Nursing Service during the war (http://www.collectionscanada.ca). Projects such as this one can be of great value to historians who can save much time, money, and effort by viewing accurate copies of original documents via their own computers.

The use of archive materials for research purposes raises a number of ethical issues—particularly relating to the confidentiality of those who produced or are referred to in the sources. Many official records are protected by law and cannot be accessed for 30 years after their production—some particularly sensitive documents are inaccessible for longer than this, often for 50 years. Such closure rules rarely apply to records relating to the history of nursing. However, concerns about the confidentiality of patient records mean that this particular type of record is rarely made available to researchers. Some hospitals may have archives that have retained some patient records, and researchers may sometimes be given access to these on condition that the names of patients are not recorded or used.

USING UNOFFICIAL ARCHIVES AND DOCUMENTS HELD IN PRIVATE COLLECTIONS

Private collections are particularly rewarding to use, but they may be difficult to access. Obtaining permission to view records that have been retained by individuals or families in their own homes can be time-consuming; care is needed. Often, these materials have been kept for very personal reasons; this may be because they are personal in nature, such as letters and diaries, or because the content is important to the way in which an individual is remembered. The fact that the family has been unwilling to send a collection of documents to an archive may indicate that they have feelings of sensitivity about its contents.

These can, nevertheless, be some of the most rewarding source materials for the historian, who may be breaking new ground in viewing material that has never been used in previous history writing. The personal contact with the owners of these documents can also add interest to the work.

USING NATIONAL LIBRARIES

National libraries are amongst the most straightforward of repositories. In developed countries they will normally have online catalogs that can be consulted in advance of a visit, their collections are very extensive, and they provide comfortable and well-lit spaces in which to work. They also share many of the disadvantages (for the historian) of archives, in that preservation may take precedence over access. Furthermore, because most of the materials available have been published in some form, issues of copyright ownership can mean that it is very difficult to obtain copies. Copyright law is complex and differs from country to country. It can often be difficult to know just how much material can be taken away and used for study purposes, and it is wise to be guided by library staff on these issues.

THE INTERPRETIVE PROCESS

A history is built on a careful examination of a range of sources. The more extensive and varied the sources, and the more angles that can be obtained on the topic under study, the better. Once the sources have been collated and read carefully, most historians will find that an interpretation begins to emerge—an argument becomes clear. It is important, however, to avoid the assumption that this is a purely intuitive process. A rigorous piece of historical research is one in which the historian remains aware of the process by which an argument was developed or a theory formed. This involves, in part, being reflective about one's own pre-existing assumptions. When writing a history, it is important to be aware of the filtration process by which the contents of the sources are channeled through one's own prejudices and presuppositions.

Any history is, of necessity, a combination of the ideas of the individuals who produced the sources on which it was built and those of the historian who mined and brought them together. In examining written and printed texts, it is useful to ask: "To what extent are these texts valid as sources? Do they have credibility? Do they convey truth?" This of course raises the further questions: "In the context of doing history, what is truth? Is it an element of fact or reality, or is it a facet of meaning, in which case, would the symbolic text be just as truthful as (if not more so than) the factual?"

These questions raise issues about the way we interpret texts. If the term *text* is taken to refer to a range of traces of the past (documents, printed sources, images, artifacts, landscapes), then the process by which historians engage with these is the essence of their work. They can engage empirically, in which case they are searching for facts (Elton, 1967; Hallett, 1997; Jupp & Norris, 1993; Mortimer, 1997; Rafferty, 1991). They can approach the text in a relativist way, in which case they are interested in how the content of the text was meaningful to its author (Carr, 1961; Hughes-Warrington, 2000). They can adopt a hermeneutic approach, which will mean that the text will be viewed as a synthesis of the perspectives or horizons of author and reader (Gadamer, 1975; Koch, 1996). If they employ discourse analysis, they will be searching for evidence of the ideological power structures that influenced the author (Schiffrin, 1994; Silverman, 1999; Titscher, Meyer, Wadale, & Vetler, 2000); and, finally, if their approach is postmodern, they will be adopting an extreme relativism, aiming to find evidence for the presence, absence, or, indeed, destruction of the great, ordering narratives that gave meaning to life (Jenkins, 1991, 1995; Southgate, 2000).

Historical work always contains within itself threats to rigor; the accuracy of the sources and the quality of the interpretation are always open to question. The interpretive approach that may counterbalance these inherent threats is the hermeneutic, in which there is a conscious attempt to give equal attention to the intentions and priorities of both author and reader (Koch, 1996; Spence, 2001). In the works of H. G. Gadamer, "hermeneutics" is presented as the most desirable of approaches because it permits the "fusion of horizons" in which the perspective of the person who wrote the text is met by the preconceptions and prejudgments of the person interpreting it, in order to produce something new that is openly acknowledged as a synthesis of the two—privileging neither one nor the other. Gadamer argues that this process is one of the "circle of understanding," in which the reader's prejudices are brought to the text and are repeatedly remodeled as the reading progresses (Gadamer, 1975).

In the 1990s, the trend in historical writing was toward increasingly relativist approaches to textual interpretation and away from what was seen as a naïve attempt to write purely empirical history (Hallett, 1997; Jenkins, 1995). Discourse analysis, in which there was an attempt to see behind the apparent content of the text to the ideological power structures of the society that had influenced its production, has remained popular amongst critical theorists (George, 2003; Traynor, 1996; Wilson, 2001). Alongside discourse analysis stood perspectives that were deliberately angled, such as feminist history (Coslett, Easton, & Summerfield, 1996; Davies, 1995; Gamarnikow, 1991; Holliday & Parker, 1997; Im & Meleis, 2001). Postmodernism, a more nihilistic approach, pervaded by an extreme form of relativism, in which there is no *History,* only *histories;* no *facts,* only *traces of the past;* and no *truth,* only a range of *perspectives* or *positions,* has been less resilient, enjoying a fairly brief period of popularity in the late 1980s and 1990s, only to lose support around the turn of the century (Foucault, 1973; Jenkins, 1995; Southgate, 2000).

CONCLUSION

Truth is a remarkably slippery concept as it appears in history; the more assertive and individualistic the writings of past authors, the clearer are their own perceptions of truth. It is profoundly difficult for the historian to define and explain truths, which appear to permeate a text, yet are not always voiced in deliberate and conscious terms.

Gadamer argued that there are two types of truth: the genetic truths, which are generated by the authors of the individual texts; and a possible universal truth, *die Sache,* which is present in all the accounts and can be elicited or extracted by the historian (Gadamer, 1975). Historical sources are mobilized by historians to support a range of arguments and lines of interpretation, rather than supporting a set of simple truths. Hence, their interpretation raises more questions than answers: Do such works constitute historical sources? Is their examination a valid endeavor for the historian?

History is an attempt to make sense of and understand the past. The same sources can be used to interpret past events in a range of different and often competing ways. In fact, it may be that the richer a source, the more competing interpretations of the past it can support. This is not to say that there are no wrong interpretations. While historians' interpretations can be valid in a range of different ways, they can also be obviously incorrect or manifestly weak. Strong history writing is marked by the care and openness with which the historian engages with their sources. It is, furthermore, characterized by a consciousness about the way in which those sources are used to support interpretation.

REFERENCES

Australian Government National Archives of Australia. (n.d.). *The collection.* Retrieved June 28, 2007, from http://www.naa.gov.au/the_collection/the_collection.html

Carr, E. H. (1961). *What is history?* Harmondsworth, UK: Penguin Books.

Collingwood, R. G. (1994). *The idea of history.* Oxford: Oxford University Press.

Coslett, T., Easton, A., & Summerfield, P. (1996). *Women, power and resistance: An introduction to women's studies.* Buckingham, UK: Open University Press.

Davies, C. (1980). *Rewriting nursing history.* London: Croom Helm.

Davies, C. (1995). *Gender and the professional predicament in nursing.* Buckingham, UK: Open University Press.

Elton, G. R. (1967). *The practice of history.* Glasgow: Fontana.

Firby, P. (1993). Learning from the past. *Nursing Times, 89,* 32–33.

Fitzpatrick, M. L. (2001). Historical research: The method. In P. L. Munhall (Ed.), *Nursing research: A qualitative perspective* (3rd ed., pp. 309–371). Boston: Jones and Bartlett.

Foucault, M. (1973). *The birth of the clinic.* London: Tavistock Publications.

Gadamer, H. G. (1975). *Truth and method.* London: Sage.

Gaddis, J. L. (2002). *The landscape of history. How historians map the past.* Oxford: Oxford University Press.

Gamarnikow, E. (1991). Nurse or woman: Gender and professionalism in reformed nursing, 1860–1923. In P. Holden & J. Littlewood (Eds.), *Anthropology and nursing* (pp. 110–129). London: Routledge.

George, J. (2003). An emerging discourse: Towards epistemic diversity in nursing. *Advances in Nursing Science, 26,* 44–52.

Hallett, C. E. (1997). Historical texts: Factors affecting their interpretation. *Nurse Researcher, 5,* 61–71.

Hamilton, D. B. (1993). The idea of history and the history of ideas. *Image: Journal of Nursing Scholarship, 25,* 45–48.

Holliday, M. E., & Parker, D. L. (1997). Florence Nightingale, feminism and nursing. *Journal of Advanced Nursing, 26,* 483–488.

Hughes-Warrington, M. (2000). *Fifty key thinkers on history.* London: Routledge.

Im, E., & Meleis, A. I. (2001). An international imperative for gender-sensitive theories in women's health. *Image: Journal of Nursing Scholarship, 33,* 309–314.

Jenkins, K. (1991). *Rethinking history.* London: Routledge.

Jenkins, K. (1995). *On 'what is history?'* London: Routledge.

Jupp, V., & Norris, C. (1993). Traditions of documentary analysis. In M. Hammersley (Ed.), *Social research* (pp. 37–51). London: Sage.

Kirby, S. (1997). The resurgence of oral history and the new issues it raises. *Nurse Researcher, 5,* 45–58.

Koch, T. (1996). Implementation of a hermeneutic inquiry. *Journal of Advanced Nursing, 24,* 174–184.

Lowenthal, D. (1985). *The past is a foreign country.* Cambridge, UK: Cambridge University Press.

Lusk, B. (1997). Historical methodology for nursing research. *Image: Journal of Nursing Scholarship, 29,* 355–359.

Maggs, C. (1987). *Nursing history: The state of the art.* London: Croom Helm.

Marwick, A. (1989). *The nature of history.* London: Macmillan.

Marwick, A. (2001). *The new nature of history: Knowledge, evidence, language.* Basingstoke, UK: Palgrave.

McGann, S. (1997). Archival sources for research into the history of nursing. *Nurse Researcher, 5,* 19–29.

Mortimer, B. (1997). Counting nurses: Nursing in the nineteenth century census. *Nurse Researcher, 5,* 30–45.

Rafferty, A. M. (1991). Historical research. In D.F.S. Cornack (Ed.), *The research process in nursing.* Oxford: Blackwell.

Rafferty, A. M. (1997). Writing, researching and reflexivity in nursing history. *Nurse Researcher, 5,* 5–16.

Schiffrin, D. (1994). *Approaches to discourse.* Oxford: Blackwell.

Silverman, D. (1999). *Interpreting qualitative data. Methods for analyzing talk, text and interaction.* London: Sage.

Southgate, B. (2000). *Why bother with history? Ancient, modern and postmodern motivations.* Harlow, UK: Pearson Education Ltd, The Longman Group.

Spence, D. (2001). Hermeneutic notions illuminate cross-cultural nursing experience. *Journal of Advanced Nursing, 35*, 624–630.

Titscher, S., Meyer, M., Wadale, R., & Vetler, E. (2000). *Methods of text and discourse analysis*. London: Sage.

Traynor, M. (1996). Looking at discourse in a literature review of nursing texts. *Journal of Advanced Nursing*, 26, 1155–1161.

Wilson, H. (2001). Power and partnership: A critical analysis of the surveillance discourses of child health nurses. *Journal of Advanced Nursing, 36*, 294–301.

CHAPTER ELEVEN

About Artifacts

Eleanor Krohn Herrmann

Artifacts are known by many names. Among them are relics, discards, collectibles, remnants, and memorabilia. Each of those terms has some element in common with the other, but none, by standard dictionary definitions, conveys the fullest possible meaning of the word *artifact.* One's own background and point of view also evoke associated meanings. Examples include nostalgia, disparagement, amazement, and appreciation (Worden, 1993). For the purpose of this discussion about artifacts (which intentionally excludes written documents because that source of data is already a recognized and accepted one), this writer believes that the following is the most encompassing, acceptable, and accurate definition. An artifact is an inanimate physical object from an earlier time, produced by human workmanship, and carried out with a view to subsequent use, but without the conscious intent of imparting connected information (Costello, 1991; Good & Scates, 1954).

Artifacts, however, have received little independent attention in the professional literature, especially as they relate to historical research. In reference to historical sources, Good and Scates in 1954 wrote that "many types of materials have not been fully utilized, especially remains or relics" (p. 182). Treece and Treece in 1973 supported that contention by stating that nursing research has left such data "relatively untouched." Inquisitively they asked, "What secrets do these data hold which could add to nursing theory and improved patient? And what contributions could they make to nurses' understanding of nursing trends?" (p. 99). The following more recent lamentation, while directed toward research in medical history, is equally applicable for historical research in nursing.

> There are wonderful opportunities for historical research in collections of medical artifacts. The challenge is getting that message across to people who have read or written about medical history without considering the artifacts and mistakenly think that they are getting the whole story. The medical artifacts themselves can often speak as powerfully as written explanations. (Worden, 1993, p. 111)

One of the immediate benefits of artifacts is the sense of continuity that is experienced when three-dimensional objects are viewed and handled. The trajectory of the development of nursing is awakened. Each artifact has its own story and invites exploration of its past while linking it to the present. An example is the evolution of "Mrs. Chase," the simplistic manikin developed in the early 1900s for teaching clinical procedures. The first Chase manikin, which was near human size and weight, could be bathed, bandaged, and positioned and receive such topical treatments as stupes and fomentations. Over the years, construction features permitted invasive actions such as injections, irrigations, catheterizations, and tracheotomy care. Consequently, the Chase doll became the prototype for the baby and the male manikins that followed. Despite the fact that all were silent and unresponsive to the care practiced on them, their legacy reflects the impact they had on generations of patients and student nurses (Bradshaw, 1986; Herrmann, 2000). Today, in the absence of the Chase manikins, there are highly sophisticated teaching models; one is called SimMan. It can simulate a host of bodily functions on command or in reaction to the nursing care practiced on him. Advances in technology and nursing's acceptance of innovations have made that evolution possible. That said, it should be acknowledged that the earliest models of SimMan are already considered out-of-date and, despite the large space required to display them, are gradually finding their way to collectors and museums. Yesterday's artifacts are tomorrow's treasures.

On another level, there is sometimes a dramatic or visceral reaction to certain artifacts. For example, upon seeing an early-1800s 14-inch-long pewter clyster, an instrument for rectal injections (Morten, 1905, p. 32), one observer exclaimed, "They used that for what? That's cruel punishment in the name of care!" Early therapeutics and current feelings can sometimes preempt the investigative process (Boraker, 1986).

A group of retired nurses had an interesting reaction to a collection of nursing artifacts. Upon seeing the artifacts, they reminisced about how they were used during their active nursing days. Further, the nurses offered previously unknown facts and foibles about the artifacts and filled in or extended knowledge about them. Shortly after the nurses returned to their homes, several packages with artifacts—ones that the collection did not already have—were received. The nurses obviously had held onto what they considered a significant part of their professional heritage—namely artifacts.

An unusual benefit of knowing about nursing artifacts was experienced by this writer while working as a nurse in a developing country. This country had limited resources, no disposable equipment, and only a few professionally prepared nurses. Therefore, this author had to work with what was available. That entailed such things as sharpening injection needles, boiling used equipment to achieve sterility, and repairing rubber gloves. Familiarity with nursing's artifacts and how they were used held the writer in good stead. Without the knowledge of nursing history and its artifacts, nursing care surely would have been compromised.

AREAS OF INQUIRY

Three questions that are frequently asked of nurse historians are: Where do you get nursing artifacts? How much can a person expect to pay for them? And, how do you determine their age? The following section of this chapter addresses those queries, along with examples and explanatory data, with the hope that the value of nursing artifacts for both teaching and research purposes will be apparent. Because there is a paucity of written information about the questions raised, particularly in a collected format, the writer has had to depend largely on her personal experience for answers. That experience includes being the founder and curator of the Dolan Collection of Nursing Artifacts at the University of Connecticut School of Nursing, completion of a certificate program at the National Archives in Washington, D.C., having served as past president of the American Association for the History of Nursing (AAHN), being a member of the board of directors of a local historic commission, and having taught both graduate and undergraduate courses in nursing history.

Acquisition

Acquisition refers to the process of obtaining artifacts, in this case, nursing artifacts. That process usually begins with ferreting out potential sources. Antique shops, flea markets, yard sales, and auctions are all possibilities, but do not expect that they will be advertised as having nursing or health care artifacts for sale. You just have to develop a discerning eye and be willing to risk being mistaken when examining or purchasing an item. An example is a purchase made by an individual who thought she had found a rare, double-spouted invalid feeder. It was a gravy separator.

And, in an antique shop known to the writer, a white enamel irrigation can, commonly used for rectal and vaginal irrigations, was labeled a "planter." Old trade and antique catalogues can sometimes provide clarity when trying to identify items. Familiarity with Herrmann's (2006) *Turn-of-the-Century Nursing Artifacts,* which is replete with illustrations and documentation, can be of further help when making choices about purchases.

Colleagues, neighbors, and friends are another potential source for artifacts. To make space for a new computer or some updated reference books, they may be happy to part with a single item or a small collection of artifacts, particularly if they know that their items will be cared for, for the benefit of present and future generations of nurses. Just make it clear that acceptance of an artifact does not necessarily ensure that it will be on temporary or permanent display.

Not to be overlooked is the disposal of about-to-be discarded health care items when new ones are being introduced. (Who ever thought that the 4" × 4" × 3" red plastic Destruclip box, a safety device used to destroy hypodermic needles and syringes, would so soon become a collectible artifact?) Also, learn about renovations that might reveal artifacts behind a demolished panel or cabinet. Do not be afraid to ask the appropriate person to alert you about such activity or to save found items until you can examine them.

Online auctions such as eBay are another source of artifacts. Diligent searching might, for example, produce a sought-after treasure such as a Nightingale-era brass and parchment lantern or a way to replace a long lost school of nursing pin, even if the school is now closed. The fact that the Internet reaches a global market is a distinct advantage. However, a concomitant drawback of this option, especially if you are buying a one-of-a-kind item, is that you cannot physically inspect it beforehand and must depend on the seller's description.

A once-in-a-lifetime opportunity to acquire artifacts arose in March 2007 when noted author and medical historian C. Keith Wilbur decided to offer his entire collection of antique medical instruments at an auction held at Skinner's Gallery in Boston. While there was a limited number of artifacts specific to nursing, the auction did include pap boats, baby feeders, a Gibson medicine spoon, and a Vapo-Cresolene vaporizer. Further, because the seller was a reputable collector, the auction left nothing in the way of questioning the authenticity of the items. Be alert for notices of such opportunities.

Another unique auction is the annual one held by the American Association for the History of Nursing (AAHN) in conjunction with its yearly conference. The AAHN provides yearly information about the conference and auction on its Web site at http://aahn.org. The majority of the items are artifacts donated and then sold with the intent of raising money for scholarships devoted to historical research in nursing. Framed artwork, glass hypodermic syringes, Cadet Nurse Corps uniforms, nursing school capes, sheet music, and invalid feeders are but a few of the many examples of artifacts sold at the auction. Heavy active bidding is characteristic of that event.

It is wise for an institution holding or developing an artifact collection to have an Acquisition Committee with policies to govern the collection. That way, decisions regarding gifts, purchases, refusals, deaccessioning, and related matters can be diplomatically and officially addressed. For example, how do you kindly say to a potential donor, "Thanks, but no thanks" when you know that you already have 10 pairs of ordinary nurses' bandage scissors, and she wants to donate her precious pair? One response might be to suggest donating the scissors to an AAHN auction.

Another consideration about acquisition relates to the scope of the collection. Will any and all nursing artifacts be accepted for the collection or will the collection have a specific focus? For example, should the artifacts be limited to a certain time period such as the American Civil War, to a geographical area such as a state, to a specialty such as home care nursing, or to leaders in nursing such as Virginia Henderson and Josephine Dolan, both of whom donated artifact collections to the University of Connecticut? Establishing parameters can be a useful way to build a coherent and meaningful collection capable of being maintained and expanded.

Determining Value

Determining the value of artifacts is both a difficult and intriguing process. One could say it is all in the eye of the beholder. Valuation entails the use of criteria specific to the item being appraised; however, the criteria vary from one field to another. For example, the criteria used to evaluate the worth of an 18th-century pewter bedpan are significantly different from those used to determine the value of a pair of handmade wooden crutches from the same era. Some appraisers refer to what they call the "trinity" when judging an artifact—rarity, beauty, and provenance. Others add that the value lies in an item's condition, importance to the field, and who once owned or was associated with the object, regardless of the object's inherent value.

Application of the latter criterion, as well as the one related to provenance, is reflected in Marguerite Manfreda's account of how and why she came into possession of the crystal necklace that Janet Geister was famous for wearing to American Nurses Association (ANA) functions. Manfreda received the necklace in gratitude for the nursing care she had given to

Geister's dying sister. Manfreda prized the crystals for many years before donating them to the Midwest Nursing History Resource Center in 1994. Both Geister and Manfreda were recognized nursing leaders. Geister had been inducted into the ANA Hall of Fame in 1984 (Manfreda, 1995). Manfreda was inducted into the Teacher's College, Columbia University Nursing Hall of Fame posthumously in 2004. Geister's necklace, passed onto Manfreda, reflected the brilliance of two prominent nursing leaders and was valued accordingly.

The difficulty in determining the value of nursing artifacts is especially true because the market for them is relatively untested. Current market prices are most often based on the rarity of the item, its condition, the purchaser's desire for ownership, and what the traffic will bear. Such things as the inclusion of an artifact's original box or set of accompanying instructions automatically demand a higher price. Even a slightly damaged artifact, if rare, will likely boost its price. Other times artifacts bring an unexplainable or unpredictable sum. Bradshaw (1986), for example, stated that she had corresponded with an antique dealer who had sold a misdated Chase hospital manikin, labeled as folk art, for $2,000.00.

Determining the Age

To begin with, one should consider the overall age rule related to artifacts. Some antiquarians say that an item must be 100 years old to legitimately qualify as an antique. Others say that 50 years is adequate. Many nursing artifacts meet both rules. However, now that nursing is very fast paced, complex, and technologically intensive, the half-century rule is increasingly becoming the standard. When it is not possible to date an artifact with absolute certainty and an approximation is acceptable, the abbreviation "c" or "ca," for circa, meaning about, may be used—for example, c.1910. Some simple-to-carry-out methods, used alone or in combination, can help in identifying the age of an artifact. The following are among them:

- Examine porcelain, pottery, glass, ceramic, or other glass items, such as the bottom rim of an invalid feeder, for use and wear marks.
- Take notice of a manufacturer's name, seal, or other identifying marks to determine, for example, the years that a factory was in operation, when the designer worked there, whether it was a domestic or foreign production, or other telling and leading clues. An item marked "occupied Japan," for instance, would reveal that it was made immediately following World War II.

- Look for a patina, the film that can gradually develop over time on some types of metal. Film on a pewter nursing bottle is an example.
- Check for chips, stains, repairs, and broken or missing parts. They often suggest heavy long-term use, as might be seen on a worn hinged instrument or the clasp on a public health nurse's bag.
- Identify the material that was used to make the artifact. Often times the material used coincided with technical and scientific advances that can be accurately dated. The evolutionary progression of bed pans is an example. First came tin, pewter, and porcelain bedpans, followed by enamel, stainless steel, and plastic–nylon ones.
- Review advertisements in professional journals and trade catalogs. In addition to promoting a particular product, an accompanying picture of a nurse in a flapper-style uniform, for example, might confirm a 1920s origin or existence of an artifact. The use of such phrases as "new and advanced" or "improved" suggest that an outdated item existed previously.

SUMMARY

A significant part of nursing's history lies in the profession's artifacts. Yet, specific information about the artifacts rarely finds its way into the literature. This chapter has addressed the value of incorporating information about nursing artifacts into historical research. Further, the chapter provided information about three areas of inquiry related to nursing artifacts—acquisition, determination of value, and determination of age. When considered in combination, the threat of historical amnesia or historical erasure can be diminished or overcome. The content of the chapter also calls to attention the need to anticipate and preserve "emerging artifacts" that are outgrowths of current and new nursing practice arenas. Nursing artifacts are inanimate objects, but when properly perceived and creatively utilized, they can significantly enliven historical research and the teaching of nursing history.

REFERENCES

Boraker, D. (1986). The syringe. *Medical Heritage, 2*(5), 340–348.

Bradshaw, M. (1986). *The dollhouse: The story of the Chase Doll.* RI: Privately published.

Costello, R. (Ed.). (1991). *Random House Webster's college dictionary.* New York: Random House.

Good, C., & Skates, D. (1954). *Methods of research*. New York: Appleton-Century-Crofts.

Herrmann, E. (2000). Connecticut nursing history vignettes: What's in a name. *Connecticut Nursing News, 73*(1), 16–17.

Herrmann, E. K. (2006). *Turn-of-the-century artifacts* (3rd ed.). Lanoka Harbor, NJ: American Association for the History of Nursing.

Manfreda, M. (1995, Spring). Janet Geister: A personal recollection. *The American Association for the History of Nursing Bulletin, 46*, 4–5.

Morten, M. (Comp.). (1905). *Nurses' pronouncing dictionary*. London: The Scientific Press.

Treece, E., & Treece, E. (1973). *Elements of research in nursing*. St. Louis: Mosby.

Worden, G. (1993). Steel knives and iron lungs: Medical instruments as medical history. *Caduceus, 9*(2), 111–118.

CHAPTER TWELVE

Ethical Guidelines and Standards of Professional Conduct

Nettie Birnbach

Ethical issues in historical research must be addressed before, during, and after one undertakes a historical investigation. Nurse historians have known this and have developed specific guidelines and standards addressing these issues. This chapter includes a reprint of *Ethical Guidelines for the Nurse Historian* (Birnbach, Brown, & Hiestand, 1993a) and *Standards of Professional Conduct for Historical Inquiry in Nursing* (Birnbach et al., 1993b). Nurse historian Nettie Birnbach, one of the authors of these two documents, introduces them with the story of their beginning. A reprint of both follows. These two documents serve nurse historians well in historical research.

BACKGROUND

In the early 1980s, a group of interested nurse historians founded the International History of Nursing Society for the purpose of sharing historical research and promoting nursing history as a suitable discipline. Based in Illinois, the Society's international title was soon deemed premature, and the American Association for the History of Nursing (AAHN) was selected as the new name for the young organization.

Annual conferences, begun by AAHN in 1984, provided an opportunity for the dissemination of historical research in nursing and a venue for networking among nurse historians. Although the annual conferences were successful in attaining their goals, little or no time was allotted for the exploration of critical issues relevant to historical research in nursing.

At the fourth annual conference in 1987, discussions among a group of nurse historians centered on the need for invitational conferences where vital issues and concerns would be addressed (J. Brown, personal communication, June 3, 2007).

The first Invitational Nursing History Conference designed to examine identified concerns was held in Philadelphia in May 1988. Among those concerns were: the quality of and funding for historical research in nursing, the integration of history into nursing curricula, and methodological issues surrounding historical inquiry. Attendees divided into four small groups, and Janie Brown was named group leader for the subject of methodological issues. One of the recommendations identified by her group centered on the need to explore ethical considerations (Lynaugh, 1988).

At the second Invitational Conference in May 1989, the group topics were narrowed to two: ethical considerations in the historical research process and integration of historical inquiry into nursing curricula. Those involved in the ethics discussion expressed the need to address ethical dilemmas inherent in nursing history research and to "consider the development of a Code of Ethics under the auspices of the AAHN" (Baer, 1989, p. 7).

Nettie Birnbach, Janie Brown, and Wanda Hiestand, as participants in the ethics group, embarked on a study of ethical codes existing among various history organizations, such as the American Historical Association, the Oral History Association, and the National Council on Public History among others. Findings confirmed the need for ethical guidelines and standards for nurses conducting historical research.

Ethical Guidelines for the Nurse Historian (Figure 12.1A) and *Standards of Professional Conduct for Historical Inquiry in Nursing* (Figure 12.1B) were produced by the three authors and shared, in draft form, with participants at the third Invitational Conference held in April 1990. Timely suggestions from the group were incorporated into the final version, and the work was copyrighted in 1991. The documents were printed in the Spring 1993 issue of the *AAHN Bulletin* along with an editorial by Janie Brown (1993). The authors believe that both documents are relevant for those conducting historical research in nursing and appreciate the opportunity to share them with a wider audience.

Ethical Guidelines for the Nurse Historian, Nettie Birnbach, EdD, RN, Janie Brown, EdD, RN, Wanda Hiestand, EdD, RN

Historians have the responsibility for interpreting the past with dedication to truth and rigorous scholarship. Explicit ethical principles should guide historical inquiry in order to assure professional competence and accountability.

I. Historians' Relationship to Sources

A. Historians work for the preservation, care, and accessibility of the historic record. The unity and integrity of historical record collections are the basis for interpreting the past.
B. Historians have the responsibility to their sources to accurately report all information relevant to the subject.
C. Historians support open access to all archival collections and the development of a database.

II. Historians' Relationship to Subjects

A. Historians have the responsibility to subjects to present historical truths insofar as they can be determined from available sources.
B. Historians at all times respect the confidentiality of their subjects. Information gained through a professional relationship must be held inviolate, except when required by law, court, or administrative order.
C. Historians must give scrupulous attention to the principles of informed consent in order to protect the rights of subjects in their research.

III. Historians' Relationship With Colleagues/Students

A. Historians share knowledge and experience with other historians through professional activities and assist the professional growth of others with less training or experience.
B. Historians acknowledge ideas of and work done by others.

IV. Historians' Relationship With the Community

A. Historians serve as advocates to protect historical resources.
B. Historians work to promote a greater awareness of and appreciation for history in schools, business, voluntary organizations, and the community at large.

Ethical Guidelines for the Nurse Historian (*continued*)

C. Historians present historical research to the public in a responsible manner.

V. Historians' Responsibility to the Canons of History

A. Historians are dedicated to truth. Flagrant manifestations of prejudice, distortions of data, or the use of deliberately misleading interpretations are abuses inconsistent with professional responsibility.
B. Historical interpretation addresses the past in all of its complexity with careful attention to the appropriate historical context.

FIGURE 12.1A *Ethical Guidelines for the Nurse Historian.*

Adapted from *Ethical Guidelines for the Nurse Historian* by the National Council on Public History. The original discussions about the need for nursing guidelines occurred in a work group at the second and third Invitational Nursing History Conferences: Critical Issues Affecting Research and Researchers (1989, 1990).

Standards of Professional Conduct for Historical Inquiry in Nursing, Nettie Birnbach, EdD, RN, Janie Brown, EdD, RN, Wanda Hiestand, EdD, RN

A. Historians' Responsibility to the Public/Community

1. Advocate for preservation of historical sources in nursing and the conservation of archival materials.
2. Promote the development of historical databases.
3. Disseminate historical findings.
4. Increase the awareness of and appreciation for the history of nursing.

B. Historians' Responsibility to Colleagues

1. Acknowledge the ideas and writings of others.
2. Promote the development of historical databases.
3. Share information/resources with colleagues to facilitate historical research.
4. Support mechanisms that assure responsible scholarship.
5. Support the work of colleagues through attendance at conferences.
6. Support the inclusion of historical research in nursing conferences.

Ethical Guidelines for the Nurse Historian (*continued*)

7. Advocate for the integration of historical research into the broader field of nursing inquiry.
8. Engage in peer review activities.
   a. Peer reviewers must have knowledge of the topical area under review.
   b. In peer review, the identity of the author must be unknown to the reviewer.

C. Historians' Responsibility to Students

1. Facilitate the mentorship role.
2. Promote student involvement in historical inquiry.
3. Foster the dissemination of historical research through existing organizations, i.e., National Student Nurses Association, Sigma Theta Tau, nursing history associations and other groups.
4. Promote the understanding of accountable behavior in research.
5. Cite students' participation in historical projects.

D. Historians' Responsibility to Subjects (Persons/Data)

1. Advocate for mechanisms that protect human subjects and data.
2. Recognize the effects of bias on subjects and the historical body of knowledge.
3. Uphold the rights of subjects to confidentiality.
4. Exercise intellectual honesty in analyzing and interpreting data.
5. Demonstrate sensitivity in the use of confidential information.

E. Historians' Responsibility to Research

1. Ascertain that resources and facilities are adequate for the scope of the research.
2. Identify prior relevant research.
3. Utilize appropriate historical research methodology.
4. Comply with all necessary legal requirements related to the data.
5. Complete the project in a timely manner.
6. Recognize the value of historical research that effectively links the past with the present and the future.

Ethical Guidelines for the Nurse Historian *(continued)*

F. Ethical Canons of Conduct in Historical Inquiry

The nurse historian shall avoid:

1. Committing plagiarism in oral or written communications.
2. Falsely injuring the reputation of others.
3. Refusing reasonable requests for resources from qualified colleagues.
4. Removing archival material, artifacts, or other historic and cultural resources from their legal repositories without prior authorization.
5. Damaging historic documents through carelessness or non-compliance with rules posted in archival agencies

FIGURE 12.1B *Standards of Professional Conduct for Historical Inquiry in Nursing.*

REFERENCES

Baer, E. D. (1989, Summer). Report on the second Invitational Nursing History Conference. *American Association for the History of Nursing Bulletin, 23*, 6–8.

Birnbach, N., Brown, J., & Hiestand, W. (1993a, Spring). Ethical guidelines for the nurse historian. *American Association for the History of Nursing Bulletin, 38*, 4.

Birnbach, N., Brown, J., & Hiestand, W. (1993b, Spring). Standards of professional conduct for historical inquiry in nursing. *American Association for the History of Nursing Bulletin, 38*, 5.

Brown, J. (1993, Spring). Editorial—Ethical considerations in historical research. *American Association for the History of Nursing Bulletin, 38*, 1–2.

Lynaugh, J. (1988, Summer). First Invitational Nursing History Conference: Critical issues affecting research and researchers. *American Association for the History of Nursing Bulletin, 19*, 8–11.

CHAPTER THIRTEEN

Using Ethical Guidelines and Standards of Professional Conduct

Sandra B. Lewenson and Eleanor Krohn Herrmann

Historians face ethical issues while doing their research. Many of these issues can be anticipated prior to the start of the study and addressed in the design. At times, however, issues arise during the study that give us pause and force us to examine our behavior. Birnbach, Brown, and Hiestand's (1993a, 1993b) *Ethical Guidelines for the Nurse Historian (Ethical Guidelines)* and *Standards of Professional Conduct for Historical Inquiry in Nursing (Standards of Professional Conduct),* reprinted in the previous chapter of this book, serve as important tools for nurse historians when examining such issues.

The *Ethical Guidelines* lists the relationships expected between the historian and their sources, subjects, colleagues, students, community, and the "canons" of history. For example, the relationship to sources encourages the "preservation, care, and accessibility of the historic record" (Birnbach et al., 1993a, p. 4). The relationship with their colleagues and students includes the expectation that historians share their knowledge and experience and recognize the "ideas of and work done" by others. The *Ethical Guidelines,* while seeming to be filled with common sense, provide a set of statements that clearly delineate the ethical way in which the nurse historian develops and maintains relationships with their work and others related to that work.

The second document, *Standards of Professional Conduct,* lists the responsibilities that historians assume when doing historical research. There is an expectation that nurse historians will behave in a responsible manner when working with the public, the community, colleagues, students, and their subjects. They also must act accordingly in respect to the "ethical canons of conduct in historical inquiry" (Birnbach et al., 1993b). Among the *Standards of Professional Conduct,* responsibilities include mentorship of students, dissemination of historical research, showing sensitivity when using the data, and in general being honest, truthful, and thoughtful in their work. This document also lists what nurse historians should avoid, such as plagiarizing, destroying historical evidence, and not playing fair.

Both the *Ethical Guidelines* and the *Standards of Professional Conduct* seem to state the obvious, but, perhaps not so obvious when faced with ethical dilemmas in historical research. These two documents offer an excellent point of reference for engaging in discussions about ethical issues. There is no one right or wrong way to behave but there may be various ways to consider ethical relationships and responsibilities in historical research. Contextual factors involved in a study, such as someone's cultural background or religious frame of reference, may alter the way nurse historians use the data or the way their subjects may want the data used. Social, political, and economic factors may also alter the decisions made about the ethical issues in a study. Nurse historians need to dialog about these possible permutations and the influence the contextual factors may have on ethical decisions that are made during historical inquiry.

USING THE GUIDELINES AND STANDARDS

In this chapter, two case studies that emanated from the experiences of nurse historians provide a starting point for a dialog about ethical issues in historical research. The cases raise questions about ethical concerns and can be used to apply the points cited in the *Ethical Guidelines* and *Standards of Professional Conduct* (Birnbach et al., 1993a, 1993b). Readers are encouraged to think beyond these two issues and whether they were handled correctly (or not). The reader is urged to think critically about these and other possible ethical issues that may arise in historical inquiry as well as to consider how to address the relationships and responsibilities one assumes as a historical researcher.

Case Study 1: Include or Not Include, That Is the Question

A hospital in a rural section of the Midwestern part of the United States was celebrating a 75th anniversary. To mark this event, the hospital contracted with a nurse historian to write the history of the hospital's school of nursing. During the study, the researcher observed that one of the nursing students she had been following in the study was missing from the official school record for a period of several months. Pursuing information about this person further revealed that the student had been pregnant. The person who she had had an affair with was a married man and a prominent leader of the institution that supported the school the student had attended.

The researcher was not sure how to deal with this new piece of information about her subject and felt that an ethical issue was at stake. Although the incident had taken place several years before, the researcher was concerned that if this information was included in the research, the family of the student could be embarrassed, as well as the institution for which the history was being written. The story about the nursing student, even though it was an interesting reflection of the time period in which she lived and may have lent an important contextual factor in the interpretation of the data, may not have served the purpose of the study. The purpose was a history to celebrate an anniversary. The researcher felt she was faced with an ethical dilemma about what to do with this information; should she include or omit it? She decided to omit this information from the study.

Case Study 2: Publish or Not to Publish, That Is the Question

In another study, a nurse historian was asked to meet with three retired nurses who had graduated sometime in the 1930s from a prestigious urban school of nursing. These women had been friends at nursing school and were now living in an assisted-living facility. They requested that the nurse historian meet with them so they could talk about their experiences in nursing school. At the first arranged meeting, the researcher spoke to one of the retired nurses, who seemed to be the gatekeeper of the group. The purpose of the interviews was discussed, and it was agreed that the interviews would not be taped, per the gatekeeper's request. The nurse historian spent time with each person, wrote careful notes, and then met again with the gatekeeper. The nurse historian was "young" in her career as a researcher, and this was her first attempt at doing an oral history. She found that after taking copious notes of anecdotal stories about what life was like in the 1930s in nursing school, she was taken by surprise when the gatekeeper asked that the stories they shared be kept private. The group, she said, did not want anything published or shared with the public because they feared that there could be retribution from some of their old faculty and administrators. They also did not want to embarrass their school with the stories they told. As a result, the nurse historian, while frustrated, felt that the data collected could not be used. The data collected over 20 years ago now sit in a file, unpublished.

THINGS TO THINK ABOUT

Be True to the Data

Simply put, be true to the data. Being true to the data, however, can be difficult and not simple at all. To be true to the data, one must know why you are doing the study and the purpose of the study. You must also know who you are and what your biases are. Your biases may influence what you would include and what you would omit, as well as the very nature of the study itself. Your responsibility as a researcher is to be self-reflective, thereby helping you clarify your thoughts. Liehr & Marcus (2002), in writing about ethical issues in qualitative research, speak about the "researcher as instrument" (p. 157). The researcher needs to "acknowledge any personal bias, interpreting findings in a way that accurately reflects participant's reality" (p. 157). This remains central to consider when dealing with historical data or participants in oral histories.

Birnbach et al. (1993a) state that historians have a responsibility to be truthful. They write that "flagrant manifestations of prejudice, distortions of data, or the use of deliberately misleading interpretations are abuses inconsistent with professional responsibilities" (p. 4). Is omitting data from the study considered a flagrant manifestation of prejudice, or deliberately misleading?

In the case studies presented, were the nurse historians true to the data? In both instances, they chose not to reveal information about their subjects. By omitting the data, did these two historians deliberately distort the interpretation? Yet, to reveal the data would have been unethical in their minds and would have violated the ethical guideline of respecting the "confidentiality of their subjects" (Birnbach et al., 1993a, p. 4).

Compounding the ethical issues in the first case study is the conflict between the historian's responsibility to the data, the relationship with the community, and the funding source for the research. The hospital expected a celebratory history of its school and may not have approved of the inclusion of the story about the affair between the student and a hospital administrator. The nurse researcher may have decided not to include the data because the data did not add to the story, or because she was accountable to the administrators who had contracted with her to write the history. Weighing the inclusion or exclusion of data requires the researcher to balance the purpose of the study and the researcher's own biases.

Know Why You Are Doing the Study

Knowing why you are doing the study is critical to the outcome of the study. For example, are you seeking a sensational look at someone's background or a scholarly critique of the past? What data do you need to include to tell an interesting and scholarly story? Birnbach et al. (1993b) write that one of the canons of ethical behavior while doing historical research includes avoiding "falsely injuring the reputation of others" (p. 5). It is the historian's responsibility to be mindful of the subject's right to confidentiality.

In the first case study, the decision to exclude information about the nursing student's pregnancy protected the reputation of the student and perhaps the reputation of the others involved. Consider the purpose of the study, which was to celebrate the institution's 75th anniversary by exploring the history of a particular school of nursing.

The *Standards of Professional Conduct* also directs us to consider who we are writing the history for, and this, too, may influence what is included. Very often the funding agency influences what is to be studied. In the example given, if the hospital that contracted with the nurse historian wanted a celebratory history, they would then not want a critic of the social or political behaviors of the past. Consider the ramifications if the information had been included. Would the interpretation of the data have been different? Would the information about the affair just serve to sensationalize the relationships between women and men in the hospital or would it depict some of the realities that nursing students may have faced in a paternalistic hospital setting?

In the second case study, the purpose of the study was to explore the life of nursing students in the 1930s. Perhaps not clarifying a broader purpose of the study may have led to the decision to deny publication of any of the material obtained during the interviews with the retired nurses. Although the researcher did not consider the stories told by the retired nurses to be "scandalous" in nature, the participants did. The participants' age and the time period in which they went to school may have contributed to their perception. They felt that revealing how they behaved on the clinical unit would be embarrassing to them and to the school.

Make Fair Judgments

Historians are responsible for making fair judgments. But, what are fair judgments? As noted earlier, knowing who you are and your biases, helps to understand what you may include or omit from the study. The ability to self-reflect enables one to be more thoughtful and aware of some of the pitfalls involved in using historical data. For example, did the inexperience of the nurse historian in the second case prevent her from perhaps rethinking the use of the data? Could she have published the stories she heard without jeopardizing the wishes of nurses who told her their stories? What benefits would have come out of publishing the stories of these retired nurses or would it have just served to sensationalize the antics they spoke of while on the hospital units? Thurgood (2002) speaks about the uniqueness of doing oral histories to uncover local stories about the development of nursing. Did we lose something in the local history of nursing when the stories were not retold?

Undergo an Institutional Review Process

Most institutions require that all research, including historical, go through an institutional review process to assure that the rights of the subjects are upheld. The institutional reviews for historical inquiry are most often an expedited process, and oral histories are "not subject to the requirements of the Department of Health and Human Services (DHHS; Application of the Department, 2007). However, it is important to go through such a step because the process itself forces one to examine the study and assure an ethical approach.

One of the standards of professional conduct for historical research in nursing asks historians to "advocate for mechanisms that protect human subjects and data" (Birnbach et al., 1993b, p. 5). The institutional review process assures the implementation of this mechanism. In the second case study, the nurse historian might have avoided the issue she faced had she gone through the exercise of an institutional review. In this instance, the nurse historian had not done so because it had not been required by the institution at the time of the investigation. She had researched the existing material on doing oral histories, but had not developed a letter of consent. Consent was verbally agreed upon by all parties. The investigator considered the retired nurses, participation in the interview as consent. Yet, even if a written consent had been used, and the participants asked the researcher to withhold the data, then the researcher would still need to consider honoring the wishes of the participants.

Review Study With Another Historian

Find someone to talk to about your study. Discuss and debate the issues that may arise or that you face during the process of the investigation. Consider when it is okay to include material and when it is not. In the case of the retired nurses, they wanted to talk and reminisce about their experiences in school but did not want their stories to be published. They felt that it was too much exposure for them. If the researcher talks about this with another historian, then the researcher may acquire another perspective on whether to publish the data or not.

Historians are responsible to "exercise intellectual honesty in analyzing and interpreting data" (Birnbach et al., 1993b, p. 5). Debating with a colleague, the data and the findings might help to clarify what needs to be included in order to be truthful to the data and respectful of the subjects. The researcher needs to be clear about their own values and must be careful about placing their own values or concerns on the subject. A colleague may be able to validate the historians' reflections and challenge them to consider various other elements in the decision-making process. While both nurse historians' decisions were not to reveal the pregnancy or the retired nurses' stories, should they have done so? How would other historians have responded had these issues been discussed before decisions were made? Working in isolation can inhibit an important dialog one may have with other colleagues engaged in similar research. Finding a forum in which to question and converse with others is an essential responsibility of a nurse historian, and yet often difficult to do.

CLOSING

This chapter is not meant to provide a theoretical discussion of ethical concerns in historical research. Nor is it meant to raise all the questions or provide answers about ethics in historical research. Rather, its purpose is to ask nurse historians to think about and raise questions about ethical issues that arise in historical inquiry. The historians in the case studies presented in this chapter felt they had handled the ethical issues in their studies as best they could, and it seemed right to them at the time. Using the *Ethical Guidelines* and *Standards of Professional Conduct,* readers are invited to think about how they would have responded to these issues and other ethical issues that may arise when doing historical research.

REFERENCES

Application of the Department of Health and Human Services Regulations for the Protection of Human Subjects at 45 CFR Part 46, Subpart A to Oral History Interviewing. Retrieved June 21, 2007, from http://omega.dickinson.edu/organizations/oha/org_irb.html

Birnbach, N., Brown, J., & Hiestand, W. (1993a, Spring). Ethical guidelines for the nurse historian. *American Association for the History of Nursing Bulletin, 38*, 4.

Birnbach, N., Brown, J., & Hiestand, W. (1993b, Spring). Standards of professional conduct for historical inquiry in nursing. *American Association for the History of Nursing Bulletin, 38*, 5.

Liehr, R. P., & Marcus, M. T. (2002). Qualitative approaches to research. In G. LoBiondo-Wood & J. Haber (Eds.), *Nursing research: Methods, critical appraisal, and utilization* (pp. 139–164). St. Louis, Md: Mosby.

Thurgood, G. (2002). Legal, ethical and human-rights issues related to the storage of oral history interviews in archives. *International History of Nursing Journal,* 7(2), 38–49.

CHAPTER FOURTEEN

Funding for Historical Research

Jean C. Whelan and Cynthia Anne Connolly

Someone once said that writing grants is like doing taxes. It can be difficult, confusing, time-consuming, and anxiety-provoking. If this is true, given that the consequences of *not* writing a grant are not as certain as not doing one's taxes (going to jail), why go through the onerous process of seeking funding to support one's historical research? A lot of nurses, however, do so and do so successfully. This chapter attempts to demystify the grant writing process and offer concrete suggestions for writing a fundable proposal.

WHY DO I NEED FUNDING?

Research support provides an important currency in the scholarly world because it demonstrates that the grantee has successfully withstood a rigorous peer-reviewed critique of the project. The funded historian dwells in the still rare world of nurse-as-primary-investigator. For the nurse historian, usually the only such scholar at their nursing school, external funding is a recognized credential that reinforces the notion that historical research is knowledge-generative research and not "fun nostalgia."

Although it may seem unfair, money also begets money. Competing successfully on the first grant enhances the likelihood that the second funding agency will look favorably on the proposal. Like the university-based nurse historian, the independent scholar also benefits from funding in that it confers prestige to acquiring editors and helps the scholar's book proposal receive attention from publishers. Furthermore, it is also necessary work because most research grants require what needs to be done anyway: tracing the research question or aims, significance, purpose, sources, methods, and setting forward a budget and timeline for completion.

Perhaps the most compelling reason for seeking funding is to obtain the indispensable financial support to carry out a research project. Most, if not all, history research projects do not require amounts of funding in the million-dollar-plus range. Yet, costs are involved in carrying out even a very small project. Obtaining a grant is the best means of securing the funds critical to carrying out a study and helps ensure the project's completion.

BEFORE YOU BEGIN

The more time spent up front organizing your project and funding goals, the less time the process will take overall. Consider the following before you begin:

1. In addition to deciding what it is you want to investigate and designing your study, consider in what way(s) your project links to a contemporary issue in nursing or health care delivery as well as the funding interests of a particular granting organization. This linkage is sometimes referred to as the "hook" and is especially important if the funding agency usually awards more direct patient care-related scholarships. If you are a beginner, attend nursing history conferences and read extensively in the secondary literature.
2. Identify the right funding sources. Search professional organizations, computerized databases, libraries, foundations, local historical societies, etc. Look for a match between the purpose of your project and the funder.
3. Figure out how much money you'll need. Will you need to travel to interview subjects or examine archival materials? Remember, duplicating archival materials is very expensive, often as high as one dollar per page. Might the project benefit from a research assistant or technical consultant?
4. Draft a timeline that includes all phases of the research and estimate additional funds to allow for unanticipated delays.
5. Ask for advice. Consult with more experienced scholars for suggestions as to how to get started and also see if they will read the final application. Contact the funding agency and speak to a representative or project officer. Inquire as to how proposals are

reviewed, what type of applications are sought, and how funding decisions are made. Find out about the average size and funding range of awards. Request a list of projects previously funded (many funding groups now list this information on their Web sites). Search out those who have been funded by the agency in the past and ask to see their applications in order to get a "feel" for how to construct your proposal.

6. The employed applicant needs to make sure there is institutional support to submit the grant. Ascertain what internal review mechanisms need to be followed as they often take time. In many instances, a project may need to be submitted to a human subjects review committee before receiving an authorizing signature, which will also take time. For example, if a grant is due May 1, a university Grants Management Office may require it submitted to them by April 15 for final review in order to obtain the necessary authorizing signatures.
7. Seek out grant-writing workshops at universities or on the Internet.
8. Many granting agencies request letters of support. Choose these individuals or organizations carefully so that the funder learns why you are the best individual to undertake this project and has the support of interested groups. For example, if you have a proposal that seeks to write a history of the American Nurses Association, a letter from the organization's president specifying access to archival materials and relevant individuals and support for the project would be essential (Box 14.1).

Box 14.1 Tips for Building a Funded Research Program

1. Start small, get seed money.
2. Obtain feedback through publication, presenting at conferences.
3. Have a "hook" for each grant application and describe how this proposed project fits with, or builds on, earlier work, clinical experience in a particular area, etc.

AS YOU WRITE

1. Have more senior scholars review and comment on drafts. Specifically invite the person to identify flaws or weaknesses, as well as

strengths. It is helpful to have presubmission reviews by those familiar with historical research and those who are not. For example, when submitting a grant to the National Institute for Nursing Research (NINR), seek advice from a nurse historian as well as a quantitative researcher familiar with NINR funding mechanisms.

2. Sell both yourself and the project in the application. Do not be afraid to let your excitement for the project come through.
3. Aim for both a specialized and a general audience. For example, define concepts such as Progressive era or the germ theory.
4. Write clearly and concisely. Wherever possible write in active instead of passive voice.
5. Emphasize the way(s) in which you have the experience and the expertise to carry out the project.
6. Concretely explain how the proposal meshes with funding agency objectives.
7. Highlight your "hook" wherever possible, reminding reviewers the way in which the proposal is unique/important/significant. How does your project fill a gap in the literature? How will the findings derived from this research influence some aspect of contemporary health care delivery? Finally, make sure you address the "so what" question, meaning that reviewers should not walk away from the application thinking that the project is interesting but has no relationship to contemporary policy or practice concerns.
8. Follow all directions and address each of the evaluation criteria. Contact the funding agency with any questions. Using section headings for each evaluation criterion forces the investigator to consider every item and makes clear to reviewers how and where these pieces of the application have been addressed.
9. Make sure all components to the application (i.e., budget, proposal, letters of support, supporting materials such as permissions from a specific archive or human subjects committee) arrive by the submission date and are clearly labeled with your identifying information (Box 14.2).

Box 14.2 Five Strategies to Help Your Proposal Stand Above the Rest

1. Make sure costs are as accurate as possible. For example, if you need to travel to Dublin, Ireland, for research, note the airline Web site from which you derived the budget for your ticket and the date you undertook the search.
2. Carefully attend to ALL formatting rules and directions.

Box 14.2 (*continued*)

3. Read and reread your proposal to make sure grammar, syntax, and punctuation are correct.
4. Avoid making self-important claims, such as "As an internationally recognized scholar in the field of..."
5. Make sure you have accounted for all relevant research/scholarship in your literature review.

FUNDING SOURCES

Whether you are an established researcher planning a major complex project, a student just beginning to learn the research process, or an independent scholar interested in a limited focused study, ample funding opportunities exist for researchers of nursing history. Funding programs are available from a wide number of public and private sources and provide varying amounts of monies for major studies as well as for smaller, less expensive projects. A good way to begin a discussion on funding opportunities is to start with a description of potential resources for focused projects.

Funding Sources for Focused Projects

Focused grants (sometimes referred to as small grants) offer a limited amount of money, generally in the $2,000–$10,000 range for a specific, time-limited project such as a 1-year study. Generally sponsored by private groups such as professional associations, libraries, or philanthropic organizations, small grants are an excellent source of funding for researchers of nursing history. In particular, the beginning researcher may find that submitting a proposal for a focused grant is a useful way to learn the grant preparation and proposal writing process.

Numerous funding sources, such as private foundations, organizations, and associations, exist and are available for historical research projects (see Box 14.3 for a partial listing of such programs). Several professional nurse organizations, such as Sigma Theta Tau International, local chapters of Sigma Theta Tau, and the American Nurses Foundation, are receptive to funding historical research. In addition, a number of organizations, as for example, the Rockefeller Archive Center, also welcome proposals that focus on nursing history. A good source of funding for focused projects are the research centers for nursing history located at universities throughout the country. These centers often award fellowships for research on nursing history (see the specific center's Web site for information).

Box 14.3 Partial Listing of Funding Agencies for Nursing History Research

American Nurses Foundation
http://www.nursingworld.org/anf/nrggrant.htm
Sigma Theta Tau International
http://www.nursingsociety.org/research/grant_small.html
Local Chapters of Sigma Theta Tau International
Contact local chapters directly
American Association for the History of Nursing
http://www.aahn.org
Center for Nursing Historical Inquiry
University of Virginia
http://www.nursing.virginia.edu/Research.cnhi.fellowship.aspx
Barbara Bates Center for the Study of the History of Nursing
University of Pennsylvania
http://www.nursing.upenn.edu/history/
National Institute for Nursing Research
http://www.ninr.nih.gov/
National Institute of Health
http://www.nih.gov
National Library of Medicine
http://www.nlm.nih.gov/grants.html
State Funding Opportunities for the Humanities
See Web sites for individual State Historical Councils and/or State Historical Associations
Federal Funding Opportunities for the Humanities
http://www.grants.gov
National Endowment for the Humanities
Complete List of Current Grant Programs
http://www.neh.gov/grants/index.html
National Endowment for the Humanities
We the People Challenge Grants
http://www.neh.gov/grants/guidelines/wtpchallenge.html
National Archives and Records Administration
http://www.archives.gov/
National Historical Publications and Records Commission
http://www.archives.gov/nhprc_and_other_grants/index.html
Rockefeller Archive Center
http://archive.rockefeller.edu/grants/

Please note that Web site addresses may change. The Web site addresses listed here reflect the most current address.

This is only a partial listing. Many more funding opportunities may be found through additional Internet and publication searches.

List Complied by Patricia D'Antonio, PhD, FAAN, RN

Grants or fellowships from foundations or associations differ from federal grants in the amount of funds available. They are generally smaller and seldom allow for salary support. Focused grants also involve a less-complex proposal-writing process than federal and other large grants.

As many research studies of a historical nature require a minimal amount of funds, small research grants are useful for a variety of projects, such as those highlighted in Box 14.4.

Box 14.4 Examples of Projects Ideal for Focused Research Grants

- Pilot projects designed to collect data that can be used to lead into larger studies.
- Supplementary funds used to augment larger projects.
- Focused studies that require a minimum of funds or time to carry out.

Many researchers combine focused research grants with larger grants to augment funds necessary for completion of a project. As no limitations exist on the number of grants to which any one individual can apply, a researcher stands a greater chance of success as the number of applications increase. Valuable experience is also gained by writing several grants. Preparing a proposal provides an excellent way to think about a study and plan out the mechanics of how a project will be carried out. Feedback and critique obtained from grant submissions is useful for future work. (Keep in mind that not all grant awarding organizations provide feedback on grants submitted.) For the researcher who is also a faculty member, obtaining a number of grants may be a necessary ingredient for promotion.

Federal Government Funding Programs

The federal government funds fellowships and grants for nurse-led studies mainly through the National Institute of Health (NIH). The NIH funds fellowships and grants on pre-doctoral and post-doctoral level as well as for more advanced researchers and established scholars.

Pre- and Post-Doctoral Fellowships and Traineeships

Pre-Doctoral Fellowships

Pre-doctoral fellowships are funded through 1 of the 27 institutes or centers comprising the NIH. The primary institute through which fellowships for nurses are awarded is the National Institute for Nursing

Research (NINR). Funding for pre-doctoral work is through the Ruth L. Kirschstein National Research Service Awards (NRSA) Training Grants and Fellowships (T32). Two types of fellowships exist on the pre-doctoral level: institutional fellowships and individual fellowships.

Institutional Fellowships

Institutional fellowship programs are awarded to eligible educational institutions and are designed as a primary means of support for graduate training. Many university schools of nursing receive training funds via the T32 funding mechanism. Pre-doctoral students enrolled in programs that hold institutional fellowship programs apply via a process as defined by the particular school of nursing.

Individual Fellowships

Individual pre-doctoral fellowships, also available through NIH, are awarded directly to an applicant. In the case of an individual pre-doctoral fellowship, the applicant submits an individual application that outlines a research plan specific to the applicant's plan of study to be carried out during the training period.

Institutional and individual NRSAs provide funds necessary to support the student's studies and research during the pre-doctoral period. This includes a yearly stipend based on annual NIH stipend levels, payment for tuition fees and health insurance, travel money for data collection and attendance at conferences, and expenses associated with the costs of research training.

Post-Doctoral Fellowships

The NIH also awards fellowships for post-doctoral training on both an institutional and individual level. As with pre-doctoral fellowships, the applicant applies either directly to the institution holding a T32 training grant for post-doctoral work, or in the case of an individual post-doctoral fellowship, directly to the specific NIH institute appropriate to the applicant's field of study. Individual post-doctoral fellowships require submitting a proposal in which the applicant outlines the training plan required to reach the goals of the fellowship. Individual and institutional post-doctoral fellowships award a yearly stipend and health insurance, pay tuition fees for courses identified as necessary to reach the goals of the training period, and provide reimbursement for travel expenses incurred as part of data collection or training activities.

Pre- and post-doctoral training fellowships supply fellows with the requisite training required to not only complete a proposed study, but also to progress and carry out future, larger studies. In the case of pre-doctoral fellowships, the outcome expected is the completion of doctoral work. Post-doctoral fellowships augment and expand research skills acquired at the pre-doctoral level. Successful completion of a post-doctoral fellowship enables the individual to assume a faculty position at a research-oriented university setting.

Benefits of Applying for a Federal Pre- or Post-Doctoral Fellowship

Applying for a federal fellowship or grant can only be described as an arduous process. Why then apply? The first and most obvious reason is to obtain funding. Graduate education is expensive. Pre- and post-doctoral fellowships supply funds not only necessary to carry out the major portions of training, but also allows some freedom from financial worries that often beleaguer students and scholars. A main objective of any researcher, particularly at the pre-doctoral level, is to create an environment in which the study can proceed with the least amount of external concerns and worries. Obtaining a fellowship will not make the applicant rich, but it does provide for much of the considerable expense of graduate education.

Aside from the financial consideration, applying for a NRSA grant is of great value for the experience obtained. Preparing a NRSA grant forces the scholar to focus on the specific aims, objectives, and purpose of the projected study and to put those items in writing. This exercise is a necessary first step for successful completion of any study. The grant-writing process requires that the applicant identify the exact purpose and aim of the study, describe the background of the study, specify the plan for carrying out the study, and explain the study's significance. A well-thought-out proposal can serve as a road map to guide the study as it progresses. Identification of any major roadblocks is made early in the process, so that the applicant can make necessary changes. For example, one of the components of any proposal is to identify data sources. If in the application process, the individual discovers that data is not available or accessible; the applicant can make alternative plans before getting too far along.

Completion of a pre- or post-doctoral fellowship proposal is an incomparable learning exercise for future researchers. It introduces the scholar to grant writing conventions used by many of the major grant- awarding institutions and organizations. Grant writing is a skill. The more one does it; the easier it becomes. Ideally, students should embark on the proposal writing process under the mentorship of an experienced researcher/sponsor. The supervision provided by a more experienced researcher supplies the beginning scholar with an opportunity to hone grant-writing skills in an advantageous way. If successful at obtaining funding, the researcher earns a well-deserved reputation as a fundable scholar.

Mentored Research Scientist Development Awards

The Mentored Research Scientist Development Award (K01) funding program is available to holders of doctoral degrees. The K01 program provides protected time for those in faculty positions for "intensive supervised career development experience" (Program Announcement, http://grants1.nih.gov/grants/guide/pa-files//pa-06–001.html). Candidates for K01 awards are individuals employed in faculty positions who are interested in obtaining research experience either new to the applicant or in which additional supervised experience is desired. The application process is similar to that of the pre- and post-doctoral fellowships (see Program Announcement for specific instructions). A K01 award provides salary support and fringe benefits and allows the awardee up to 75% of protected time for research activities.

Federal Grant Programs for Established Scholars

For those who have completed doctoral study and are ready to embark on large-scale major research projects, an ideal source of funds for historians of nursing is the National Library of Medicine's Grants for Scholarly Works in Biomedicine and Health (G13). The G13 program is equivalent to, and carries the same prestige as, the RO1 awarded by the NINR and other NIH Centers. The Grant for Scholarly Works in Biomedicine and Health program is open to faculty and established

Box 14.5 A Few Caveats Regarding NIH Grants

- NIH grants are available only to U.S. citizens; noncitizen nationals, that is, individuals from U.S. possessions such as American Samoa; and permanent residents of the United States.
- All NIH grant programs use standardized applications that must be submitted electronically.
- The NIH maintains a very informative Web site from which detailed instructions can be accessed. In addition, each institute has an expert and very helpful staff who are available for assistance.
- Submission dates for NIH grant applications occur periodically throughout the year and are found on the NIH Web site.
- With the exception of predoctoral fellowships, NIH grants are available to holders of doctorate degrees only.

scholars affiliated with institutions capable of sponsoring the grant. Applicants complete a proposal process available through the NLM (see NLM Web site). In general, the G13 funding program provides funding for book completion projects. Grants are also awarded for electronic publications such as Web sites. G13 grants provide funds for salary support, expenses incurred as a result of work entailed in data collection, costs of travel to conferences, and other expenses. Grants are awarded for 1 to 3 years.

A number of other agencies fund large studies and are available to researchers of nursing history. (See Box 14.3 for a partial listing.) Information specific to each program can be obtained directly from the program. Many of these agencies may be unfamiliar with the current state of the body of knowledge of nursing history and the significance and potential impact of nursing history research. As more and more researchers of nursing history apply for grants from major funding sources, the more recognized nursing history becomes. It is also important to keep in mind that all funding agencies, including the NIH, change funding priorities from time to time. Areas of research that are sought one year may not be so fundable the next year. The savvy researcher keeps well-informed and up-to-date on funding priorities by regularly checking the agency's Web site and talking with agency staff about any changes (Box 14.5).

State Funding Sources

Many state or local historical societies provide funding for historical studies. This is a potentially rich source of funds for nurse researchers, particularly for those scholars who examine state and local nursing issues. Information concerning such programs can be obtained by contacting the organization directly.

THE GRANT PROPOSAL PROCESS

After making the decision to submit a proposal for a research project and choosing the funding agency to which to submit the proposal, the investigator begins the submission process. The submission process involves putting the proposal together, sending the proposal to the funding agency by the due date, and awaiting the results. It is important for the investigator to keep in mind that funding agencies adhere strictly to the specified proposal submission date. Late applications are not accepted. Investigators need to make sure they initiate the proposal writing process in plenty of time to complete and send the final proposal by the due date.

The wait time between submitting a proposal and receiving the results varies from a few weeks to, in the case of federal grants, as long as 9 to 12 months. Estimates of award notification dates can be found in the grant-application instructions.

While each funding organization has an application process unique to its own requirements, all grant proposals contain similar parts. In general there are five main components to any research proposal:

- Research plan
- Projected budget
- Curriculum Vitae or biosketch
- Letters of support
- Appendixes

Research Plan

The research plan is designed to tell the reviewers what the study intends to accomplish, describes how the study will be carried out, identifies the existing data for the study and how that data will be handled, and highlights the significance of the study. Variations exist in the format of each particular research plan, yet, all research plans include six general sections: an abstract, the project aims or objectives, a section describing the background and significance of the project, a description of prior work completed on the project, time frame for completion of the project, and a bibliography.

The research plan is the component of the proposal in which the investigator spends the greatest amount of preparation time. It is in the research plan that the investigator sells the funding agency on the project. For success, it is essential that writing skills must shine throughout the plan. It is also critical that the plan makes a good deal of sense to the reviewers and that the investigator convinces the reviewers that the study is worthy of funding. Investigators want to convey to the proposal reviewers that the study will make an important contribution to nursing knowledge, that the study is eminently doable, and that the investigator possesses the abilities to carry out the project. A good research plan is focused, coherent, logical, compelling, and convincing.

Projected Budget

Putting an estimated budget for a research project together sometimes appears to be a daunting task. In reality, creating a budget is a fairly straightforward activity. The first consideration in developing a budget is to determine what expenses are allowable according to the terms of the grant. Only allowable items as outlined in the grant instructions should be included in the budget.

Once the investigator decides what expenses to request, estimates of cost are calculated. Several practical guidelines exist to use in determining reasonable amounts to request. The most important ingredient to developing a budget is that the estimates of costs are reasonable, based on identified standards, and are justifiable.

Some grants, in particular federal grants, award both direct and indirect costs. Direct costs are those involved in carrying out the study. Indirect costs are funds paid to the sponsoring institution (generally the academic institution in which the investigator is employed) for expenses involved in sponsoring the study. In determining the amount of indirect costs, investigators should use the resources and staff of their home institution's grant management office.

The grant management office of the investigator's employing institution can provide assistance not just with determining direct and indirect costs, but also in helping to prepare the entire budget. Investigators should involve staff of the grant management office early in the grant-writing process. Staff are often valuable resources and can assist in expediting the final compilation and submission of the grant.

Items to be Considered in a Budget

Salary Support

For grants that provide salary support, the investigator should use the current salary received as the base salary from which to make estimates of salary support requested. The amount of salary support is frequently determined on a level of effort basis. For example, if it is determined that 30% of the investigator's time will be spent on the project and the investigator's salary is $60,000 a year, then the salary support will be calculated as $18,000. (The federal government currently uses the level of effort calculated as "person months." See http://grants.nih.gov/grants/policy/person_months_faqs.htm#q1 or contact the specific NIH program directly for further information.) The percent effort should be based on a reasonable estimation and expectation that the investigator will be expending the stated amount of effort on the project.

For grants that run for more than 1 year, salary estimates for each year of the grant should include a yearly increase, based on the employing institution's general rate of salary increases. Some grants, such as grants awarded by NIH, also include the cost of fringe benefits as part of salary support. Estimates of the amount of fringe benefits to include can be calculated based on the employing institution's regular fringe benefit rate.

Travel Expenses

Archival collections are often located at a distance from the researcher's home, so travel expenses for data collection activities comprise a major part of the budget for historical studies. In the case of focused grants, travel expenses may comprise the total amount of requested funds. Some grants, such as those sponsored by NIH, also allow for inclusion of expenses related to attendance at professional conferences.

Travel expenses include the costs of travel to the particular site, meals and lodging, and incidental expenses, such as necessary phone expenses. A good resource to use for estimating travel expenses is the Federal Government's General Service Administration's (GSA) travel Web site (http://www.gsa.gov/Portal/gsa/ep/home.do?tabId=0). This Web site provides per diem rates for locations throughout the United States and internationally as well as a breakdown of standard rates for hotels, meals, and incidental expenses. The GSA rates can be used as a standard for estimating travel costs for both federal and nonfederal grants. For train and airfare travel, the investigator can use typical airline and train rates for travel to the particular location as found on the airline and train Web sites. The cost of automobile travel is generally based on a rate per mile. The GSA mileage reimbursement rates for automobile travel can be used to estimate costs for trips by car.

Supplies

Supplies include paper supplies, mailings, copying expenses, and books necessary to carry out the research. In some cases, the costs of items such as electronic equipment may be permitted. Funding agencies will have specific policies regarding such costs.

Research Assistance

Funding agencies may allow for the cost of hiring research assistants. Research assistants can be valuable assets in carrying out certain projects. If affiliated with a university or college, the investigator can estimate the cost of research assistance based on the general hourly rate used by the institution.

Consultants

Consultants may be required for specific projects. For example, a project that involves statistical expertise that the primary investigator may not possess, may require hiring an expert. Consultant fees are generally estimated at the usual and customary rate charged for the consultation.

Budget Justification

Inclusion of a justification for each expense listed is a typical component of a budget. Even if the funding agency does not ask for a justification, it is a good idea to provide one. The justification explains the reasons behind asking for the expense and describes how the investigator determined each amount. For example, in the case of travel expenses, the investigator would explain that overnight travel for a certain number of days is required to a specific location for data collection purposes and that the cost of such travel was estimated using standard rates as found in the GSA Web site.

During the course of carrying out the study, the investigator will be required to submit receipts and a log of actual travel expenses to receive reimbursement. Researchers should develop an organized system of keeping a record of expenses as the study proceeds.

Some agencies offer fellowships that may not require inclusion of a specific budget. In this situation the investigator receives a set amount of funds awarded for the fellowship. If that is the case, the investigator should still maintain meticulous and accurate financial records of how the award was spent during the course of the study. This avoids confusion in the event of any questions raised later. Maintaining reliable financial records also provides the investigator with a history of how grant money was used. A record of expenses on one project can be referred to as a guide for future projects.

Curriculum Vitae or Biosketch

Funding agencies will ask the investigator to include either a Curriculum Vitae (CV) or biosketch as part of the grant proposal. This provides the funding agency and grant reviewers with information on the career history of the investigator. In many cases the funding agency will specify exactly what is to be included in this section. For example, NIH uses a very specific form for biosketches with very detailed instructions on what to include. Content included on the CV or biosketch should provide background information helpful to the reviewers and that highlights areas that focus on the qualifications necessary to carry out the study. As with all other components of the proposal, include only areas for which the funding agency specifically asks.

Letters of Support

Letters of support are statements of recommendation obtained from experts, mentors, colleagues, and faculty that testify to the investigator's skills and ability to carry out the proposed study. Letters of support let the reviewers know the opinions of others with whom the investigator has worked and provides an idea of the strengths the investigator brings to the research project. A good letter of support includes an appraisal of both the intended project as well as an assessment of the investigator's ability to carry out the project. Letters of support should be solicited from individuals who are known not only to the individual investigator, but are also well known in the field of study. An investigator, particularly a new investigator, may not be readily known to reviewers, but a letter of support from a leading figure on the topic to be studied lets the reviewers know that, in the referee's estimation, the project is worthy and the investigator capable. Solicit letters of support early in the process and provide the referee appropriate documentation, such as a copy of the proposal and a CV or biosketch to familiarize the referee with the specifics of the project. Follow the funding agency's specific directions regarding sending letters of support to the agency. In some cases, the agency requests that letters of support are sealed or sent directly to the agency; in other cases, the investigator includes the letter with the proposal.

Appendixes

Appendixes to a grant include items such as a writing sample, an instrument to be used as part of the study, informed consents if required, or other miscellaneous materials. Only include an appendix if the instructions allow.

SENDING THE PROPOSAL

Once the proposal is completed, the investigator should make a final review to ensure that all components are included and that the proposal is ready for submission. More and more funding agencies use an electronic submission procedure. If that is not the case, follow the instructions for submitting the proposal via mail and include the specified number of copies requested. Include a cover letter with the proposal.

If You Are Not Funded

1. Allow yourself a few days to be disappointed, but do not despair. You have received practice writing a proposal and framing your work for a particular audience.
2. Seek advice from a mentor or funder and try again.

If You Are Funded

1. Remember you will need to do project reports at regular intervals to keep the funding agency apprised of your progress. Make sure you keep organized financial records while you're doing the work so that you will be able to account for all of the funds awarded.
2. Sometimes funds need to be reapportioned during the project. For example, if you budgeted travel to an archive and later decide that the trip is not needed, the funds for that portion of the project cannot automatically be spent on other items. Almost always, the investigator must request approval to "rebudget" expenses.
3. Congratulations! Get to work, and have a great time!

APPENDIX ONE

Artifacts: Additional Resources

Eleanor Krohn Herrmann

Bennion, E. (1979). *Antique medical instruments.* Berkeley: University of California Press.
This resource is heavy with images and descriptions about the various antique medical artifacts.

Congdon-Martin, D. (1991). *Drugstore and soda fountain antiques.* Westchester, PA: Schiffer.
This book, with full-color photographs and informative text, includes items that nurses and the public used in the past to heal illness and soothe aches and pains.

Herrmann, E. (2006). *Turn-of-century nursing artifacts* (3rd ed.). Lanoka, NJ: American Association for the History of Nursing.
This unique monograph provides images of nursing artifacts as well as documentary sources for each.

Historical Museum of Medicine and Dentistry. (1979). *A catalogue of selected items.* Hartford, CT: Author.
A slim catalogue that presents selected items important to the history of medicine and dentistry.

Sandelowski, M. (2000). *Devices and desires: Gender, technology, and American nursing.* Chapel Hill: University of North Carolina.
A scholarly presentation with emphasis on gender, technology, and American nursing.

Warner, D. (1994). *Old medical and dental instruments.* Buckinghamshire, UK: Shire.
In a selection labeled "domestic items," a limited number of Victorian items are presented that could be reclassified as "nursing items."

Wilbur, C. (1997). *Revolutionary medicine, 1700–1800* (2nd ed.). Guilford, CT: Glove Pequot Press.
In a review published by the *Journal of the History of Medicine and Allied Sciences,* this book was described as "a pleasant and stimulating introduction to a very complicated and important subject... a delightful and much needed work."

Wilbur, C. (2000). *Antique medical instruments* (4th ed.). Atglen, PA: Schiffer.
Although the title of this book suggests otherwise, many of the numerous beautifully hand-drawn images reveal the evolution of nursing care items.

Zwelling, S. (1985). *Quest for a cure: The public hospital in Williamsburg, Virginia, 1773–1885*. Williamsburg, VA: The Colonial Williamsburg Foundation.
This book, through its narrative and pictures, provides insight into the early methods of treatment for persons with "insane and disordered minds."

APPENDIX TWO

Nursing History Centers, Museums, and Archives

Janet L. Fickeissen

INTRODUCTION

The following appendices (Appendices Two and Three) containing Internet resources are from the American Association for the History of Nursing, Inc. Web site (www.aahn.org). While it was current at the time of printing, Web sites are subject to reorganization at any time. If a listing does not work, the reader should try these strategies:

- Go to the AAHN Web site
- Go back in the directory to the root, for example, if www.aahn.org/features/posters.html does not work, try www.aahn.org/features/
- Use a search engine

This is a listing of some centers and archives available for study of the history of nursing. It is not a comprehensive list; historical research involves considerable searching for source material. But this list includes regional centers that serve as nursing repositories and some specialty nursing organizations with archives as well as institutions with significant holdings in nursing. Additional collections may be found within organizations, agencies, and universities.

Following are some archive databases for collections in the United States. These may be accessed through subscription or a library.

ArchiveGrid provides access to detailed archival collection descriptions. Access is through subscription or agencies: www.archivegrid.org/

ArchivesUSA: archives.chadwyck.com/, provides access to an integrated database of three major information resources:

- NUCMC—National Union Catalog of Manuscript Collections,
- NIDS—National Inventory of Documentary Resources in the United States, and
- DAMRUS—Directory of Archives and Manuscript Repositories in the United States.

The National Union Catalog of Manuscript Collections (NUCMC), Library of Congress, also has a searchable database: www.loc.gov/coll/nucmc/

Internet Archive is a nonprofit that was founded to build an Internet library with the purpose of offering permanent access for researchers, historians, and scholars to historical collections that exist in digital format: www.archive.org/

The History of the Health Sciences Section of Medical Library Association has a list of History of the Health Sciences Libraries and Archives: www.mla-hss.org/histlibs.htm

NURSING HISTORY CENTERS, ARCHIVES, AND MUSEUMS WITHIN THE UNITED STATES

American Association for Nurse Anesthetists (AANA) Archives

This association's archives provides references concerning the history of nurse anesthesia and the AANA.

222 S. Prospect Ave.
Park Ridge, IL 60068-4001
www.aana.com

American National Red Cross

The Hazel Braugh Records Center houses current and inactive records of the American National Red Cross and has a collection of books, photographs, tapes, and films.

American Red Cross
5818 Seminary Road
Falls Church, VA 22041
Tel: (703) 813-5380

Fax: (703) 813-5389
www.redcross.org/museum/exhibits/braugh.asp

Many historical American Red Cross nursing files are in the Red Cross gifted material at the National Archives (II), managed as Records Group 200. Indexes to this material are available at both the Hazel Braugh Center and the National Archives:

National Archives II at College Park
8601 Adelphi Road
College Park, MD 20740-6001
Tel: 301-713-6800

For World War I Era Military Nursing, records are located at National Archives (I). For a Guide to Federal Records in the National Archives of the United States see: www.archives.gov/research/guide-fed-records/

Pennsylvania Avenue at 7th Street, NW
Washington, DC 20408
Tel: 202-501-5385
www.archives.gov/

Archives of Nursing Leadership

The Archives of Nursing Leadership is a joint program of the University of Connecticut School of Nursing and the Thomas J. Dodd Research Center. The archives acquires, preserves, and makes accessible the papers and records of Connecticut organizations that support the nursing profession and the personal papers of individuals who have made a significant contribution to nursing within the state. The collection includes the Josephine Dolan papers, the Virginia Henderson Research Collection, the Connecticut Training School for Nurses Alumni Association, and the North East Organization for Nursing (NEON). The extensive collection of nursing artifacts is displayed in the School of Nursing for study and research purposes.

Archives & Special Collections
Thomas J. Dodd Research Center
405 Babbidge Rd U-205
University of Connecticut
Storrs, CT 06269-1005
Tel: 860-486-2524
www.lib.uconn.edu/online/research/speclib/ASC/findaids/Dolan/MSS19950028.html#d0e32

Barbara Bates Center for the Study of the History of Nursing

The Center, at the University of Pennsylvania, was established in 1985 to encourage and facilitate historical scholarship on health care history and nursing in the United States. The Center continues to create and maintain a resource for such research; to improve the quality and scope of historical scholarship on nursing; and to disseminate new knowledge on nursing history through education, conferences, publications, and interdisciplinary collaboration.

University of Pennsylvania School of Nursing
318R Claire M. Fagin Hall
418 Curie Boulevard
Philadelphia, PA 19104-9959
Tel: 215-898-4502
E-mail: NHistory@pobox.UPenn.edu
www.nursing.upenn.edu/history/

Bellevue Alumnae Center for Nursing History

The Center is a part of the Foundation of the New York State Nurses' Association. Some of the holdings are:

- NYSNA, New York State Nurses for Political Action, Records, 1971–1987
- New York State School Nurse Teachers Association, Records, 1931–1978
- NYSNA 1952–98, Genesee Valley Nurses' Association Archives, Records, 1939–1945
- Ellis Hospital School of Nursing
- New York State Nurses for Political Action
- New York State School Nurse Teachers Association
- Nurses Association of the Counties of Long Island Archives, Records, 1920–1991
- District 1 of NYSNA, Records, 1919–1969
- Council of Deans of Nursing: Senior Colleges and Universities in New York State, Records, 1964–1993
- Nurses House Archives, Records, 1925–1998
- "Preserving the History of Psychiatric/Mental Health Nursing: A Guide to Locating Psychiatric/Mental Health Nursing Records in New York State"

Bellevue Alumnae Center for Nursing History
The Veronica Driscoll Center for Nursing
2113 Western Avenue
Guilderland, New York 12084-9501
Tel: 518-456-7858 ext. 24
Fax: 518-452-3760
www.FoundationNYSNurses.org

Center for Nursing Historical Inquiry

Established at the University of Virginia in 1991 to support historical scholarship in nursing, the Center is dedicated to the preservation and study of nursing history in the United States. The goals of the Center include the collection of materials, the promotion of scholarship, and the dissemination of historical research findings. The Center runs a regular series of nursing history forums, sponsors the annual Agnes Dillon Randolph Award and Lecture, mounts exhibits, awards a yearly historical research fellowship, and publishes a newsletter, *Windows in Time.*

University of Virginia Health Sciences Center
McLeod Hall
University of Virginia, Charlottesville
Charlottesville, VA 22903
Tel: 434-924-0131
E-mail: nurs-hxc@virginia.edu
www.nursing.virginia.edu/centers/history.html

Center for Nursing History, Ethics, and Human Rights

The Center for Nursing History, Ethics, and Human Rights, established at Purdue University in 2003, promotes leadership and advocacy in historical, ethical, and human rights issues influencing health care.

Center for Nursing History, Ethics, and Human Rights
Purdue University School of Nursing
502 N. University Street
Johnson Hall of Nursing
West Lafayette, IN 47907-2069
Tel: 765-494-4023
Fax: 765-494-6339
www.nursing.purdue.edu/centersandclinics/cnhehr/

Clendening History of Medicine Library

The collection includes letters from Florence Nightingale, which have been digitized.

University of Kansas Medical Center
3901 Rainbow Blvd
Kansas City, KS 66160-7311
Tel: 913-588-7244
Fax: 913-588-7060
clendening.kumc.edu/

Crile Hospital Archives

This is a former U.S. Army Hospital that has both a museum and archives.

The Crile Archives Western Campus CCC
11000 Pleasant Valley Road
Parma, OH 44130
Tel: 216-987-5594
Fax: 216-987-5050
www.crile-archives.org/

History of Medicine Division at the National Library of Medicine

The National Library of Medicine manuscript collection includes the American College of Nurse Midwives, the Henry Street Settlement, National Organization for Public Health Nursing, the Society of Superintendents of Training Schools, the National League for Nursing Education, and the National League for Nursing.

The Prints and Photographs Collection includes a pictorial documentation of nursing; an index is available and copies may be purchased.

History of Medicine Division, National Library of Medicine
8600 Rockville Pike
Bethesda, MD 20894
Tel: 301-496-5405
www.nlm.nih.gov/

Historical Nursing Archives of Westchester/Rockland County [NY] Lienhard School of Nursing, Pace University

This collection focuses on local nursing history in Westchester/Rockland Counties, New York, emphasizing the activities of schools of nursing and health care organizations. The collection has five major categories: Zeta Omega at-Large Chapter of Sigma Theta Tau International; Nurses Association of Westchester County of New York State; Lienhard School of Nursing, Pace University (NY); New York Medical College Graduate School of Nursing; and miscellaneous photographs, artifacts, books, audio-visual tapes, and other materials. A finder's guide is available online; please call for an appointment.

The collection is housed on the Pleasantville Campus of Pace University in the Doris and Edward Mortola Library:

861 Bedford Road
Pleasantville, New York, 10570
Tel: 914-773-3380
www.pace.edu/historicalarchives

Mary L. Pekarski Collection in the Burns Library, Boston College

The Pekarski Collection has focused on the history of nursing, bioethics, and the Catholic, especially Jesuit, influence on nursing. The collection includes: Josephine Dolan Collection, including letters from Florence Nightingale and Dorothea Lynde Dix; the New England Deaconess Hospital School of Nursing Collection, from founding in 1893 to closing in 1989; the Rita P. Kelleher Collection; the Margaret Colliton Collection; MICA; VNA of Boston; Legal/Ethical Aspects of Nursing; The American Association of Nurse Attorneys; and North American Nursing Diagnosis Association (NANDA) archives.

www.bc.edu/libraries/centers/burns/

Midwest Nursing History Research Center

The Center's museum with artifacts is in the Nursing School at the University of Illinois, Chicago.

845 S. Damen Ave.
Chicago, IL 60612-7350
Tel: 312-996-0621
Fax: 312-996-8945
E-mail: ghlo@uic.edu
www.uic.edu/nursing/ghlo/resourcecenter/index.shtml

Records and papers have been moved to the University of Illinois at Chicago University Archives at the Library of the Health Sciences Special Collections Department.

Archives/Special Collections
Library of the Health Sciences
University of Illinois at Chicago
1750 West Polk
Chicago, IL 60616-7223
Tel: 312-996-8977
www.uic.edu/nursing/ghlo/resourcecenter/index.shtml

Museum of Nursing History

The museum is an important educational arm for the community concerning the contribution of nursing past and present. It is a repository in which individuals can place priceless memorabilia—books, documents, letters, photographs, scrapbooks, yearbooks, caps and uniforms (prior to 1920), medals, pins, and military artifacts.

Friends Hospital
8th & 4641 Roosevelt Blvd.
Philadelphia, PA

Museum's Mailing address:
The Museum of Nursing History, Inc.
761 Sproul Road, #299
Springfield, PA 19064
Tel: 215-843-9501
www.nursinghistory.org/index.htm

The Florence and Ike Sewell Museum, Northwestern Hospital, Chicago

Student nurse uniforms, caps, pins, and other nursing memorabilia are displayed in the Florence and Ike Sewell Museum.

Northwestern Hospital
251 East Huron Street
Feinberg Pavilion, 3rd Floor
www.nmh.org/nmh/forhealthcareprofessionals/nurse_scrapbook.htm

History of Nursing Archives

Established in 1966 with help from a U.S. Public Health Service grant and the support of the Boston University School of Nursing, the History of Nursing Archives contains the personal and professional papers of nursing leaders; records of the schools of nursing; public health and professional nursing organizations; histories of various American and foreign schools of nursing, including early textbooks; as well as a very extensive book collection. These manuscripts and books document the evolution and contribution of the nursing profession in the fields of public health and military history.

Howard Gotlieb Archival Research Center
Boston University
771 Commonwealth Avenue
Boston, MA 02215
www.bu.edu/archives/holdings/historical/nursing.html

Oncology Nursing Society Archives

The primary focus is association records as well as history of nursing oncology.

Oncology Nursing Society
501 Holiday Drive
Pittsburgh, PA 15220-2749
Tel: 412-928-9584 #255
Fax: 412-921-6565
www.ons.org/publications/library/

Rush University Medical Center Archives

These Chicago nursing schools have their records at Rush:

- Presbyterian Hospital School of Nursing
- St. Luke's Hospital Training School for Nurses
- Presbyterian-St. Luke's Hospital School of Nursing
- Rush University Medical Center Archives

1700 West Van Buren Street, Suite 086
Chicago, IL 60612
Tel: 312-942-7214
Fax: 312-942-3342
www.lib.rush.edu/archives/

Southern Labor Archives

Located in the Special Collections Department at Georgia State University. The collections include records of state nurses associations from the District of Columbia, Maryland, Kentucky, South Carolina, Georgia.

Special Collections & Archives
Georgia State University Library
100 Decatur Street SE
Georgia State University
Atlanta, Georgia 30303-3202
www.library.gsu.edu/spcoll/pages/area
asp?ldID=105&guideID=510

Southwest Center for Nursing History

Part of the Center for American History at the University of Texas at Austin, the focus of this collection is regional nursing organizations.

University of Texas School of Nursing
1700 Red River
Austin, TX 78701
Tel: 512-471-4910
www.lib.utexas.edu/taro/utcah/00366/cah-00366.html

University of Maryland School of Nursing Museum

Permanent museum exhibition and growing archives documenting the evolution of Maryland's largest and oldest continuously operated school of nursing from its founding as a hospital training school in 1889 to a leading research institution. Museum transcends its institutional roots to offer an evocative depiction of modern American nursing.

University of Maryland School of Nursing Museum
655 W. Lombard Street
Baltimore, Maryland 21201
Tel: 410-706-1502
Fax: 410-706-0399
nursing.umaryland.edu/offices/development/museum/index.htm

U.S. Army Center of Military History, Army Nurse Corps Collection

This Web site contains considerable content and photographs relevant to the history of the U.S. Army Nurse Corps.

Army Nurse Corps Historian
Office of Medical History, Office of the Surgeon General
5109 Leesburg Pike
Falls Church, VA 22041
Tel: 703-681-2849
history.amedd.army.mil/ANCWebsite/anchhome.html

ViaHealth Archives Consortium

The Baker-Cederberg Museum and Archives, Genesee Hospital Archives, TGH School Nursing Archives, Myers Community Hospital, Sodus, New York, Rochester General Hospital collects and preserves materials and disseminates information that chronicles the development of Rochester City/Rochester General Hospital and its affiliates. The collections include the School of Nursing at Rochester City/General hospital (1880–1964); Isabella Graham Hart School of Practical Nursing (1964–present); Florence Nightingale Post American Legion (1918–present); Base Hospital 19 (1916–1920); 19th General Hospital, AUS (1940–1950); Fitch's French Military Hospital (1914–1919); Genesee Hospital; Myers Community Hospital; Behavioral Health (Rochester Mental Health Center) Collection; plus several tenant collections including: the New York State and Genesee Dietetic Associations and the Society for Total Emergency Programs (STEP)

ViaHealth Archives Consortium
333 Humboldt Street
Rochester, NY 14610
Tel: 585-922-1847
www.viahealth.org/body_rochester.cfm?id=331

CANADIAN ARCHIVES AND CENTERS

Archive Databases for Collections in Canada

Archives Canada provides access to online resources

www.collectionscanada.ca/

Guide to Canadian Nursing Archival Resources, from Canadian Association for History of Nursing:

www.cahn-achn.ca/pdf/Archival%20Resource%20Guide.pdf

Canadian Centers and Museums

Associated Medical Services Nursing History Research Unit

The AMS Unit is the first funded research unit in Canada dedicated to the history of nursing. The Research Unit will develop, nurture, and coordinate the study of nursing history in Canada.

The Unit also aims to coordinate the donations of nursing archival sources to appropriate depositories and to maintain a comprehensive bibliography on Canadian nursing history. The AMS Nursing History Research Unit is located in the School of Nursing at the University of Ottawa, Ontario, Canada.

Room 3245A, School of Nursing
University of Ottawa
451 Smyth Road
Ottawa, ON K1H 8M5
Canada
Tel: 613-562-5800 Ext. 8424
www.health.uottawa.ca/nursinghistory/index.htm

Margaret M. Allemang Centre for the History of Nursing

The Margaret M. Allemang Centre for the History of Nursing is an organization open to anyone interested in the history of nursing in Ontario, Canada. Founded in 1993, the Centre works to increase the visibility of nursing's major role in our society. The archival goal of the Centre is to locate, collect, and preserve archival resources related to the history of nursing in Ontario and make accessible such resources. Their newsletter is online.

355 Millwood Road
Toronto, Ontario M4S 1J9

Canada
www.allemang.on.ca/archives.html

Musee des Hospitalieres de l'Hotel-Dieu de Montreal

Located next to the Hotel-Dieu Hospital, this museum tells the story of the foundation of Montreal and of the exceptional life of Jeanne Mance. Although not a member of the order, she led the work of cloistered nuns who tended the sick in early Montreal beginning in 1644.

201 Avenue des Pins Ouest
Montreal, Quebec H2W 1R5
Canada
Tel: 514-849-2919
www.museedeshospitalieres.qc.ca/

Nursing History Resource Centre

The Nursing History Resource Centre was established in July 1992 through the initial support of the Nurses Association of New Brunswick. The Centre, custodian for New Brunswick nursing's past, has an exhibit area that holds display cases with pin and cap collections, nursing tools, medical artifacts, pictures, and uniformed mannequins. An adjoining archive holds collections of nursing books, scrapbooks, audio-visual artifacts, catalogued pictures, primary and secondary source documents, and so forth.

Nurses Association of New Brunswick
165 Regent Street
Fredericton, NB E3B 7B4
Canada
Tel: 506-458-8731
Fax: 506-459-2838
www.nanb.nb.ca

INTERNATIONAL

Archive Databases for Collections Outside the United States and Canada

ARCHON

Directory includes contact details for record repositories in the United Kingdom.

www.nationalarchives.gov.uk/archon

Archives Hub

A national gateway to descriptions of archives in UK universities and colleges.

www.archiveshub.ac.uk/index.html

Register of Australian Archives and Manuscripts (RAAM)

www.nla.gov.au/raam/

New Zealand National Register of Archives and Manuscripts (NRAM)

www.nram.org.nz/

UNESCO Archives Portal

An international gateway to information for archivists and archives users.

www.unesco.org/cgi-bin/webworld/portal_archives/cgi/page.cgi?d=1

EAN: European Archival Network

www.european-archival.net/

International Archives and Centers

Documentation Centre for Nursing / Hilde-Steppe-Archive (Germany)

Located in Frankfurt, Germany, The Documentation Centre started with the personal collection of Hilde Steppe. While the current focus is nursing during the Nazi era, it is hoped that it will be possible in the future to expand the collection of the Centre to include other important aspects of German and European nursing history.

Mailing address:
Fachhochschule Frankfurt am Main
Dokumentationsstelle Pflege / Hilde-Steppe-Archive
Nibelungenplatz 1
60318 Frankfurt am Main, Germany
www.hilde-steppe-archiv.de/

Institute for the History of Medicine of the Robert Bosch Foundation

In 1994, the Robert Bosch Foundation launched a grant program for projects on the history of nursing. Since then, nursing history has become one of the main research fields of the Institute for the History of Medicine (www.igm-bosch.de), complementing the two other areas of research, social history of medicine and history of homeopathy. The Institute organizes national and international congresses and workshops.

It also keeps enlarging its research library by buying books on nursing history. The Institute cooperates with the Ruhr University of Bochum in collecting nursing history sources from the German-speaking countries.

Straussweg17
D-70188 Stuttgart, Germany
www.igm-bosch.de/

Danish Museum of Nursing History

The museum is housed in a former sanitarium for children with tuberculosis. A library and an archive are also housed here.

Fjordevej 152
Strandhuse, 6000 Kolding, Denmark
www.dshm.dk

Florence Nightingale Museum Trust

The Museum is located at St Thomas Hospital, London.

2 Lambeth Palace Road,
London SE1, 7EW UK
Tel: 00 44 20 7620 0374
Fax: 00 44 171 928 1760
www.florence-nightingale.co.uk

The Royal British Nurses' Association Archives

Minutes from 1887, membership records, other organization archives are housed at King's College, Kings's College, The Strand, London, WC2R 2LS.

To use the archives contact the RBNA:

Riverbank House Business Centre, Room 502
1 Putney Bridge Approach
London SW6, 3JD UK
www.r-bna.com/archives.asp

Royal College of Nursing, Scotland—Archives and Oral History Collection

The RCN Archives are a unique record of the development of the profession of nursing in the United Kingdom. Founded in 1916, the archives record its role as a professional organization with international links, as an educational body providing the first post-registration courses for nurses in the United Kingdom, and as a trade union negotiating, lobbying, and campaigning. The RCN Archives hold the records of other nursing organizations and of hundreds of individual nurses in its oral history collection.

RCN Archives
42 South Oswald Road
Edinburgh EH9, 2HH UK
Tel: 0131 662 1010
E-mail: archives@rcn.org.uk
www.rcn.org.uk/resources/historyofnursing/collections.php

Royal College of Nursing Archives

The RCN Archives aim to record and preserve materials relating to the professional and social history of nursing and to provide a research resource for scholars and the public.

42 South Oswald Road
Edinburgh, EH9 2HH UK
Tel: 0131 662 1010
Fax: 0131 662 1032
www.rcn.org.uk/resources/historyofnursing/collections.php

UK Centre for the History of Nursing

The UK Centre for the History of Nursing is a joint venture between The Royal College of Nursing (RCN) and Edinburgh's Queen Margaret University College (QMUC) that provides a focus for nursing history in Europe. Both RCN and QMUC have outstanding archive and educational resources that are the heart of the Centre. Its task is to build awareness of the importance of nursing history through education and research. The Web site has links to archival material in the United Kingdom.

www.ukchnm.org/

Welcome Library

Collections of books, manuscripts, archives, films, and pictures on the history of medicine from the earliest times to the present day. There is a significant collection of Nightingale material in this collection and a Guide to Nightingale Sources at Welcome Library is available online: library.wellcome.ac.uk/assets/wtl039832.pdf

183 Euston Road
London NW1 2BE
library.wellcome.ac.uk/

APPENDIX THREE

Nursing History Internet Sites

Janet L. Fickeissen

The following appendice containing Internet resources are from the American Association for the History of Nursing, Inc. Web site (www.aahn.org). While it was current at the time of printing, Web sites are subject to reorganization at any time. If a listing does not work, the reader should try these strategies:

- Go to the AAHN Web site
- Go back in the directory to the root, for example, if www.aahn.org/features/posters.html does not work, try www.aahn.org/features/
- Use a search engine

The following are some of the many Web sites with nursing history content.

100 Years of Nursing Caps From Canadian Museum of Civilization

www.civilization.ca/hist/infirm/inint01e.html

Ad*Access

Ad*Access Project, funded by the Duke Endowment "Library 2000" Fund, presents images and database information for over 7,000 advertisements printed in U.S. and Canadian newspapers and magazines between 1911 and 1955. Nurses appear in hygiene ads and World War II ads.

scriptorium.lib.duke.edu/adaccess/

Adventures of Red Cross Nurses During Franco-Prussian War of 1870

Adventures of Red Cross Nurses in the 1870 Franco-Prussian War, the 1876 Serbo-Turkish War, and in battles with the first chairman of the British Red Cross. Emma Maria Pearson and Louisa Elisabeth Maclaughlin were two of the earliest Red Cross nurses, and their experiences staffing field hospitals are recounted and annotated by G. Harry Mclaughlin, Louisa's great-nephew. There are links to three separate publications.

www.harrymclaughlin.com/LouisaMcLaughlinFirstRedCross Nurse.htm

A History of U.S. Army Base Hospital No. 48—Nurses

This page is part of the Homéopathe International, a French non-profit organization dedicated to develop an information database on homeopathy on the net.

homeoint.org/books2/ww1/48nurses.htm

American Nurses Association Centennial

The professional organization for nurses celebrated their centennial in 1997, and some of the history is presented on this site.

www.nursingworld.org/centenn/

American Nurses Association Hall of Fame

The ANA Hall of Fame pays tribute to distinguished nurses in our past. A brief biographical sketch is available.

nursingworld.org/hof/index.htm

American Association for the History of Medicine

The AAHM Web site has links to many interesting resources in the history of science and medicine.

www.histmed.org/

American Collectors of Infant Feeders

For those who collect nursing artifacts, specifically invalid feeders, this is a collectors' organization. The ACIF considers invalid feeders a "go-with" or related item. Their Web site has information on both the association as well as the history and information on invalid feeders, pap boats, medicine spoons, and similar items.

www.acif.org/

American Historical Association

Home page for the American Historical Association.

www.historians.org/

An 1895 Look at Nursing

Reproduced at this Emergency Nursing World site is a very long excerpt from the book *Ambulance Work and Nursing—A Handbook on First Aid to the Injured With a Section on Nursing, Etc.* W. T. Keener & Co. circa 1895.

www.enw.org/1895_Nursing.htm

Archives for Research on Women and Gender (ARWG)

ARWG is under the direction of the University of Texas—San Antonio. This Web site provides not only the Women's Archives of Texas but provides links to women's archival collection throughout the country and a few international collections as well.

lib.utsa.edu/Archives/WomenGender/

Army Nurse Corps Association

ANCA is a voluntary organization of, by, and for U.S. Army Nurse Corps officers.

www.e-anca.org/

Black Nurses in History

This is a "bibliography and guide to web resources" from the UMDNJ and Coriell Research Library. Included are Mamie O. Hail, Mary Eliza Mahoney, Jessie Sleet Scales, Mary Seacole, Mabel Keaton Staupers, Susie King Taylor, Sojourner Truth, and Harriet Tubman.

www4.umdnj.edu/camlbweb/blacknurses.html

Brief History of Black Women in the Military

This feature was written by Kathryn Sheldon, former Curator for Women in Military Service for America Memorial Foundation, Inc.

www.womensmemorial.org/Education/BBH1998.html

Canadian Association for the History of Nursing (CAHN)

Founded in 1987, the CAHN is an interest group of the Canadian Nurses Association with the purpose to promote interest in the history of nursing and to develop scholarship in the field. Their annual meetings are in June.

www.cahn-achn.ca/

The Caps Collection in the Nursing Museum on the Web UW-Madison

The caps collection in the Nursing Museum of the University of Wisconsin, Madison, features caps from nearly 100 schools of nursing.

www.son.wisc.edu/alumni/history/historical_collections/hist_collections.html

Cherry Ames

This site has an extensive collection of material related to the *Cherry Ames* series. Included is the essay "Cherry Ames War Nurse: Fiction Meets Reality" and complete lists of the books in this series, as well as links to other nurse books, such as the Miss Pinkerton series written by (nurse) Mary Roberts Rinehart.

www.netwrx1.net/CherryAmes/

Civil War

There are a staggering number of Civil War sites. The following are relevant to nurses.

"The Angels of the Battlefield": www.civilwarhome.com/civilwarnurses.htm
Army Nurses in the Civil War: www.edinborough.com/Learn/cw_nurses/Nurses.html
National Museum of Civil War Medicine: www.civilwarmed.org/
Women and the Civil War, Inc.: womenandthecivilwar.org/index2.htm

Country Joe McDonald's Florence Nightingale Tribute

This site contains a chronology of Nightingale and is loaded with images. Unfortunately there is poor documentation, although he mentions Sir Edward Cook's biography of Miss Nightingale. There is also a lovely calendar that can be printed out.

www.countryjoe.com/nightingale/

Edith Cavell

This is one of many resources on Edith Cavell on the Internet.

www.edithcavell.org.uk

Ethel Bedford Fenwick University of Sheffield

Mrs. Bedford Fenwick was a significant figure in the history of British nursing. There is a feature and biography on the site.

www.shef.ac.uk/~nmhuk/adltnur/people/fenwick.html

Frontier Nursing Service

On this site is a brief history of the midwifery service founded by Mary Breckinridge in 1925. The page is by Kentucky Coalition of Nurse Practitioners and Nurse Midwives.

www.frontiernursing.org/History/History.shtm

History Matters

Created by the American Social History Project/Center for Media and Learning (Graduate Center, CUNY) and the Center for History and New Media (George Mason University). There are many stories of nurses and nursing here—use the keyword search.

"This Is How It Was": An American Nurse in France During World War I
Beyond Bedpans: The Life of a Late Nineteenth Century Young Nurse
"Cutting a New Path": A World War II Navy Nurse Fights Sexism in the Military
Kellogg African American Health Care Project: The Oral Histories

Also on this site is *Making Sense of Evidence,* guides to primary source material.

historymatters.gmu.edu/d/60

History of Health Sciences Resources

This jump site for resources in all health sciences is from the Web site for the History of the Health Sciences Section of Medical Library Association.

www.mla-hhss.org/histlink.htm

History of Medicine On-Line

An online journal devoted to the history of medicine.

www.priory.com/homol.htm

Hospital Ship International

John Gilinsky created this Web site about hospital ships from all over the world. There are some links to sites with historical information about hospital ships.

www.geocities.com/Athens/Forum/2970/

History of HIV/ AIDS

To commemorate the 20th anniversary of the first publication about AIDS, The NIH History Office launched a Web site, *In Their Own Words: NIH Researchers Recall the Early Days of AIDS.* The Web site features some of the oral history interviews the NIH Historian Victoria A. Harden and her colleagues have done since 1988 with NIH physicians, scientists, nurses, and administrators whose work comprised the NIH's response to AIDS between 1981 and 1988.

aidshistory.nih.gov

History of Medicine Resources

Selected Special Collections and Archives in the History of Medicine from Yale's Cushing/Whitney Medical Library.

info.med.yale.edu/library/historical/speccoll.htm

History of Registration, from Rochester, NY

The Nursing Practice Act—The Armstrong Act of 1903 was the third in the United States. This Web site, from ViaHealth Archives Consortium in Rochester, NY, describes the passage of the bill.

www.viahealth.org/body_rochester.cfm?id=516

History of Registration, from Royal British Nurses' Association

Ethel Bedford-Fenwick, the mover and shaker for registration in the United Kingdom, is featured on this site.

www.r-bna.com/registration.asp

Library of Congress: American Memory from the Library of Congress Historical Collection for National Digital Library

American Memory consists of collections of primary source and archival material relating to American culture and history. These historical collections are the Library of Congress's key contribution to the national digital library. Most of these offerings are from special collections of the Library of Congress (lcweb.loc.gov/spcoll/spclhome.html)

rs6.loc.gov/amhome.html

Also available from the Library of Congress is material on Walt Whitman, including his "Hospital Notebook."

memory.loc.gov/ammem/collections/whitman/

Margaret Sanger Papers Project

Margaret Sanger, birth control activist, was a nurse. This Web site details the project of the Department of History at New York University to arrange and publish her papers, which are in the Sophia Smith Collection at Smith College Archives. Information about video productions and links to related Web sites are available.

www.nyu.edu/projects/sanger/

MedHist

Sponsored by the Wellcome Library for the History and Understanding of Medicine [UK], this is a guide to history of medicine resources on the Internet.

www.intute.ac.uk/healthandlifesciences/medhist/

MedWeb

Another site that provides numerous links to health history resources on the Internet is the history section of MedWeb, which is maintained by Emory University Health Sciences Center Library.

www.medweb.emory.edu/MedWeb/

Internet Modern History Sourcebook

There are some source materials to be found here, including Florence Nightingale on Rural Hygiene, from *Selected Writings of Florence Nightingale*. But the site also has material on studying history and using primary sources.

www.fordham.edu/halsall/mod/modsbook.html

My Aunt My Hero

Helen Fairchild was a member of the Pennsylvania Hospital Unit during World War I. This Web site features a summary of her life and considerable correspondence from Miss Fairchild to family during her service at the front.

www.vlib.us/medical/MaMh/MyAunt.htm

My Mother's War

Helen T. Burrey was an American nurse who served as a Red Cross Nurse during World War I. She documented her experience in both a journal and a scrapbook, which has been treasured by her daughter, Mary Murphy. Ms. Murphy has placed many of these items on the Internet for people to access, and it provides a firsthand account of that experience. Additionally, she has a variety of links to other WWI resources.

www.murphsplace.com/mother/main.html

National Archives and Records Administration (NARA)

The Archival Research Catalog (ARC) is the online catalog of NARA's nationwide holdings in the Washington, DC, area Regional Archives and Presidential Libraries. Most of the holdings related to nurses are military nurses.

www.archives.gov/research/arc

National League for Nursing (NLN)—History

This page offers a brief history of the NLN at three points in the last century: from its start in 1893 as the Society for Superintendents of Training Schools, the reorganization and name change in 1952, and some contemporary activity.

www.nln.org/aboutnln/info-history.htm

National Library of Medicine—Online and Digital Exhibits

A selection of their collection is online.

www.nlm.nih.gov/onlineexhibitions.htm

Native Women Veterans

This page, by Brenda Finnicum, started as a tribute to and history of Native American Nurses in the Army Nurse Corps. It has expanded to include all Native American women veterans.

www.nativewomenveterans.org

Navy Nurse Corps: Oral Histories, Corps History, and Photographs

Oral Histories from Navy Nurse Corps are online as well as some photographs and history.

www.history.navy.mil/faqs/faq50-1.htm

New Haven's Hospitals

This is the first of Yale's Historical Library's online Tercentennial exhibits. It features photographs and ephemera related to the origins, early years, and complex interactions of the city and their relations to Yale University.

info.med.yale.edu/library/exhibits/hospitals/

Nursing History Links—Nurses.Info

Nurses.info is owned and financially sponsored by Australian Nursing Agency. There are some pages on nursing history and links to other sites.

www.nurses.info/history.htm

The Nursing Museum on the Web—UW-Madison

There is a collection of articles on nursing history here, including "The Cadet Nurse: The Girl With a Future."

www.son.wisc.edu/alumni/history/historical_collections/hist_collections.html

Historical Nursing Journals Database—Royal College of Nursing

Historical nursing journals database has digitized *The Nursing Record* to facilitate and promote research into the history of nursing by improving access to early nursing journals. *The Nursing Record* was published from 1888 to 1956, changing its name in 1902 to *The British Journal of Nursing*. The RCN Archives catalogue is also available.

www.rcn.org.uk/resources/historyofnursing/historicaljournals.php

The Nursing Sisters of Canada

A history of nursing sisters of Canada from Veterans Affairs Canada.

www.vac-acc.gc.ca/general/sub.cfm?source=history/other/Nursing

Nova Scotia Nursing History Digitization Project

This site explores the history of nursing education in Nova Scotia from 1890, when the Victoria General Hospital established the first nursing school in Nova Scotia, to the late 20th century. The development of the nursing schools are explored by integrating narrative text with photographs and documents from the schools.

www.msvu.ca/library/archives/nhdp/

Pioneer Nurses of West Virginia

Linda Cunningham Fluharty has developed this site that explores history of nurses, schools, and hospitals in West Virginia.

www.lindapages.com/nurses/nurses.htm

Online Images From the History of Medicine

This system provides access to nearly 60,000 images (reproducing photographs, artwork, and printed texts) drawn from the extensive collection of the History of Medicine Division at the U.S. National Library of Medicine. This database is searchable; this is a very busy Web site.

wwwihm.nlm.nih.gov

Queen Victoria and Florence Nightingale

From Royal Insight, an exhibit on Queen Victoria and the Crimea.

www.royal.gov.uk/output/Page3944.asp

Rockefeller Archive Center

The Rockefeller Archives, located in Tarrytown, NY, has a significant collection related to nursing *and* funding is available for researchers using their collections.

archive.rockefeller.edu/

Schlesinger Library on the History of Women in America, Radcliffe College

Archives and women's history center.

www.radcliffe.edu/schles

Sigma Theta Tau International—Heritage Committee

This has information on the role of an archival consultant by Veronica C. O'Day and a list of the Heritage Committee, which is meant to assist STTI chapters in preserving their history.

www.nursingsociety.org/chapters/arch_role.html

Southern Association for the History of Medicine and Science

They hold an annual conference in the spring.

www.sahms.net

U.S. Army Nurse Corps—History

The U.S. Army Nurse Corps is rich in nursing history, and this Web site has much of that history.

history.amedd.army.mil/ANCWebsite/anchhome.html

AN Historian & Deputy Chief
Office of Medical History, Office of the Surgeon General
Skyline 5 Suite 401B (Attn DASG-MH)
5109 Leesburg Pike
Falls Church, VA 22041-3258

Virginia Nursing History

Virginia Nursing History was compiled by the Joint History Committee of the Virginia Nurses' Association and the Virginia League for Nursing and is maintained by Special Collections and Archives, Tompkins-McCaw Library, VCU Libraries, Virginia Commonwealth University.

www.library.vcu.edu/tml/speccoll/nursing/index.html

Visiting Nurse Service of New York—History

Where it all began with Lillian Wald, Mary Brewster, and the Henry Street Settlement. Their history is presented by Karen Wilkerson, PhD, RN and Shirley H. Fondiller, EdD, RN.

www.vnsny.org/mainsite/about/a_history.html

Women's History Resources

These Web sites provide links to many resources on Women's History.

National Women's History Project: www.nwhp.org/
Women's History: A Todd Library Research Guide: frank.mtsu.edu/~kmiddlet/history/women.html

Women in Vietnam

This Web site has a collection of articles and published documents, including letters and audiotapes by and about women who served in Vietnam. There are also links to the Virtual Wall for each nurse who died in Vietnam.

www.illyria.com/vnwomen.html

Index